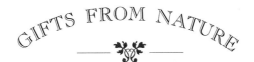

# GIFTS FROM NATURE

# LOTIONS, OILS AND ESSENCES

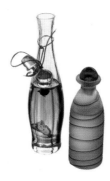

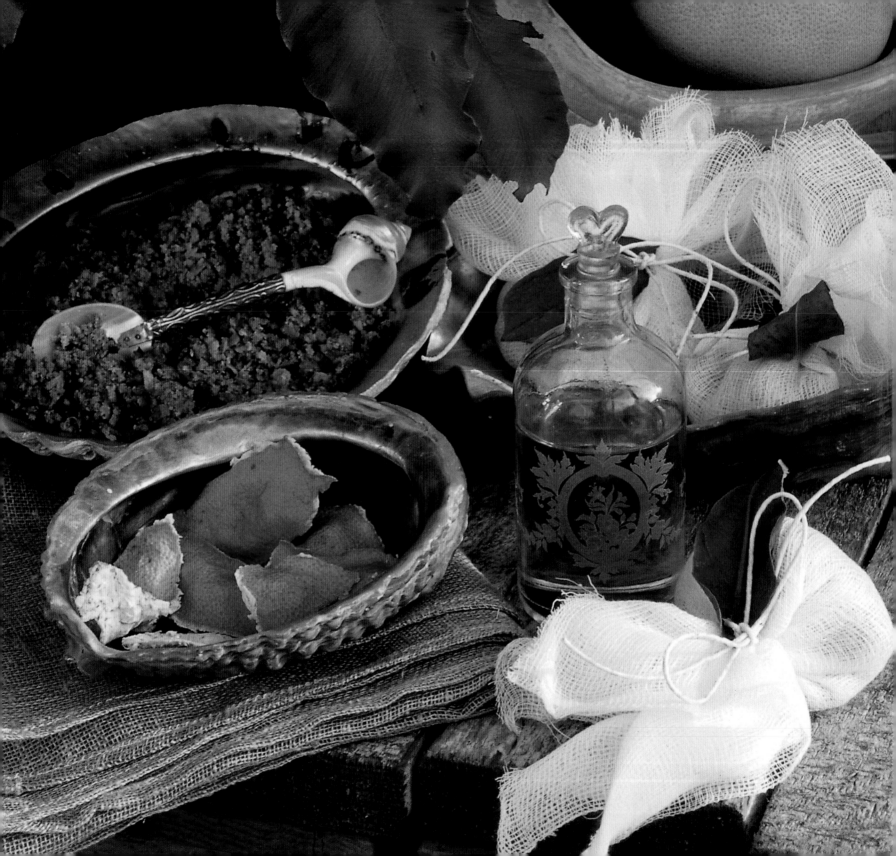

# GIFTS FROM NATURE

# LOTIONS, OILS AND ESSENCES

Bathroom and beauty products from natural ingredients

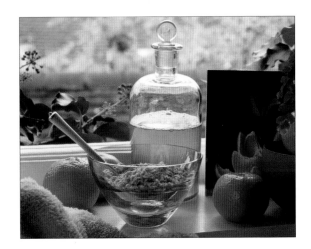

JOANNE RIPPIN

LORENZ BOOKS

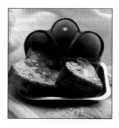

This edition first published in 1998 by Lorenz Books

© Anness Publishing Limited 1998

Lorenz Books is an imprint of
Anness Publishing Limited
Hermes House
88-89 Blackfriars Road
London SE1 8HA

This edition distributed in Canada by
Raincoast Books
8680 Cambie Street, Vancouver
British Columbia V6P 6M9

ISBN 1 85967 591 3

A CIP catalogue record for this book is available from the British Library

Publisher: Joanna Lorenz
Project Editor: Joanne Rippin
Designers: Lisa Tai and Lilian Lindblom
Illustrations: Anna Koska

Printed and bound in Singapore

1 3 5 7 9 10 8 6 4 2

# CONTENTS

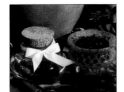
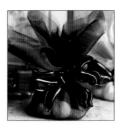

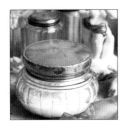
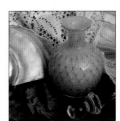

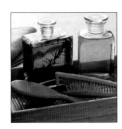
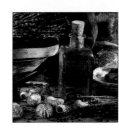

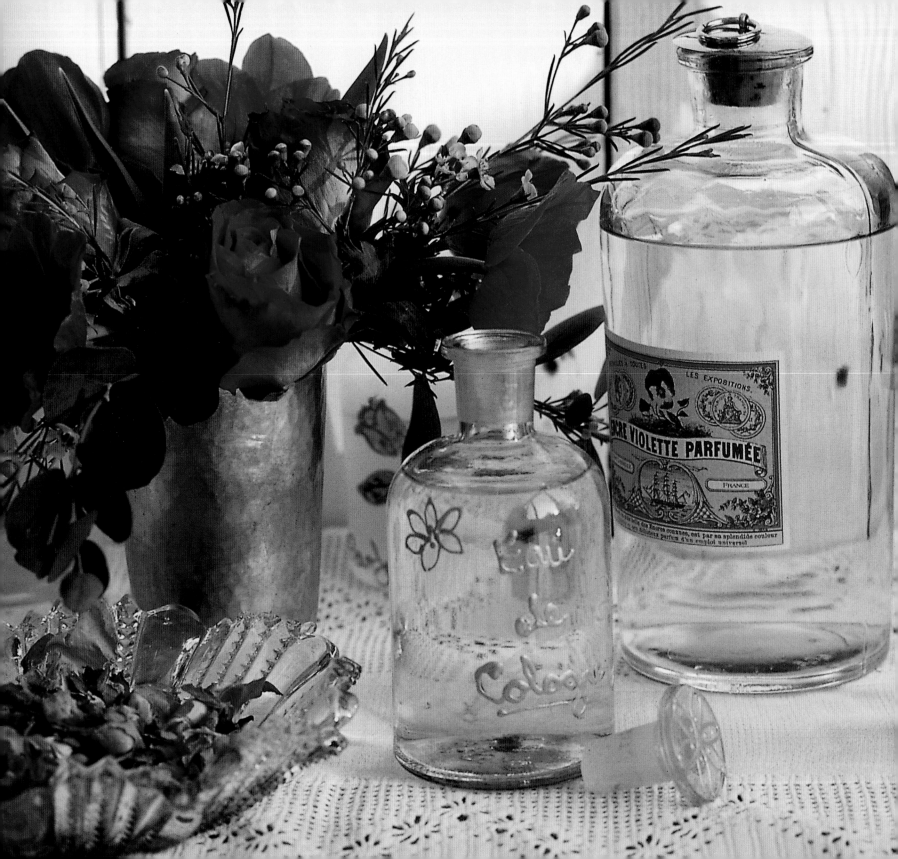

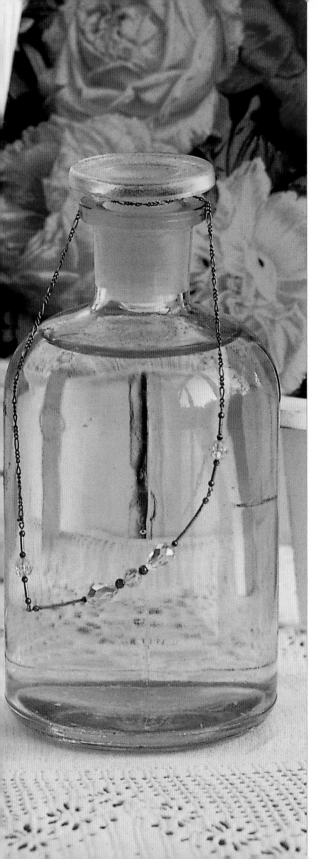

# INTRODUCTION

*W*e have grown so used to buying beauty treatments and skin care products that we tend to forget how simple it can be to prepare them ourselves. There are dozens of highly effective treatments, many of them traditional, that you can make at home, usually at a fraction of the price you might pay in the shops.

In addition, home production allows you to ensure that the ingredients are the best and as pure as possible. You can use organically grown herbs and flowers and bottled water to avoid harmful chemicals coming in contact with your skin. Buy essential oils from a reputable company as they vary greatly in quality. Although all the ingredients used in these recipes are safe, it is advisable to do a patch test with any new cream or lotion before using it on your skin or hair. Spread a small amount on your inner arm and leave it for 24 hours to see if you develop an allergic reaction such as a rash.

Scales, a measuring jug and a set of spoons will enable you to measure the ingredients accurately. Keep this equipment separate from cooking utensils as any residues of oils and waxes may taint your food. You will also need a double boiler for melting waxes, as direct heat could burn them. Store lotions and creams in china or coloured glass containers to protect them from light that can harm the oils; essential oils can migrate into plastic.

These beauty formulas are all easy to concoct and make lovely gifts when presented in pretty bottles or jars. As they are free of preservatives, home-made cosmetics need to be kept in the fridge: include this advice on a label if they are intended as gifts.

# CLEANSING AND PURIFYING

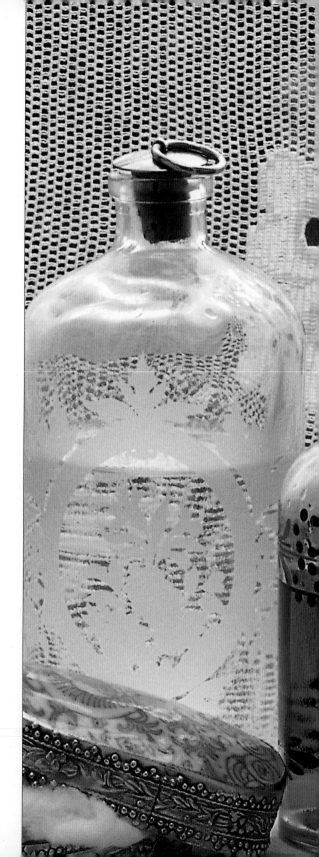

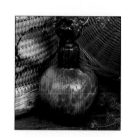

Simple home-made cleansers for the skin and hair have been tried and found reliable for hundreds of years. The beneficial effects of clay and oatmeal, for instance, were known by the ancient Egyptians. Masks and scrubs using traditional ingredients like these leave the skin clean and revitalised. Alternatively, you can add your own ingredients to unscented soap. Hairdressers recommend using

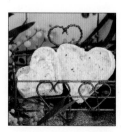

a variety of treatments to keep hair looking its best, and in this chapter you will find a range of herbal hair rinses to try. Both fresh herbs and essential oils can be used to improve hair and scalp health.

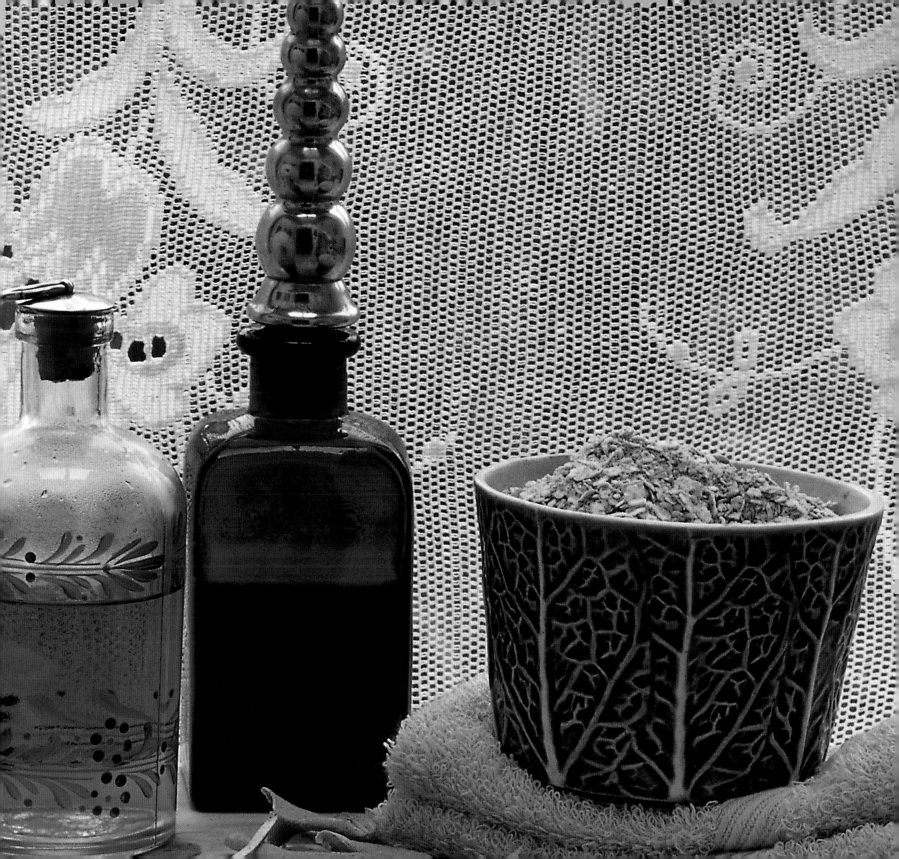

# Fennel cleanser

---❦---

*Made in minutes, this cleanser can be used daily to lift grime gently away.*

- 15 ml/1 tbsp fennel seed
- pestle and mortar
- 250 ml/8 fl oz/1 cup boiling water
- strainer

- 5 ml/1 tsp honey
- 30 ml/2 tbsp buttermilk
- spoon
- stoppered glass bottle

**1** Lightly crush the fennel seeds using the pestle and mortar. Pour on the boiling water and allow to infuse for 30 minutes.

**2** Strain the liquid, then stir in the honey and buttermilk. Pour the cleanser into a clean stoppered bottle and keep it in the fridge.

# Soapwort cleanser

---❦---

*This gentle, foaming liquid cleanser is ideal for sensitive skins.*

- 15 g/½ oz chopped soapwort root (available from herbalists)
- small stainless steel or enamel saucepan
- 600 ml/1 pint/2½ cups bottled water

- unbleached paper coffee filters
- mixing bowl
- 50 ml/2 fl oz/¼ cups rose-water
- spoon
- 600 ml/1 pint/2½ cups stoppered glass bottle

**1** Place the soapwort root in the pan, pour in the water, bring briefly to the boil, then leave to simmer for 15 minutes.

**2** Strain the liquid through coffee filter papers until it is clear. Stir in the rose-water, then decant into the bottle.

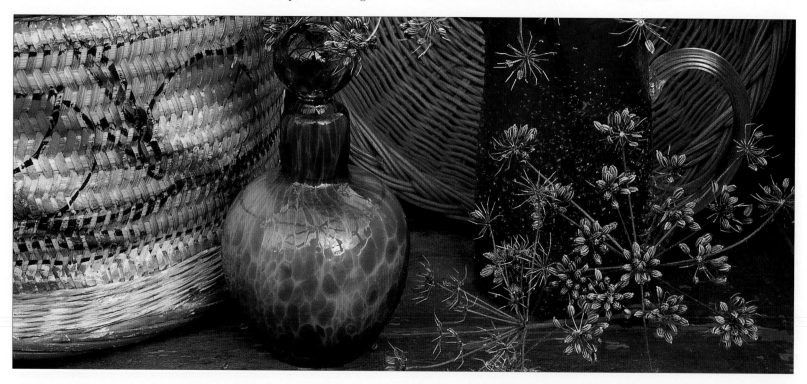

# ROSE CREAM CLEANSER AND FACE MASK

*This mildly astringent cleanser has soothing and cooling qualities. The face mask is suitable for dry skin but gentle enough for sensitive faces. Adding oatmeal produces a mask that can also be used as an exfoliating skin scrub. The mask is most effective if used on the face and neck while you are lying in the bath. Wash it off thoroughly after about 10 minutes.*

**Cleanser**
- 105 ml/7 tbsp triple-distilled rose-water
- 45 ml/3 tbsp double cream

**Face mask**
- 5 ml/1 tbsp triple-distilled rose-water

- 45 ml/3 tbsp double cream
- 30 ml/2 tbsp pure unblended clear honey, gently warmed
- 30 ml/2 tbsp fine ground oatmeal (optional, for face scrub)

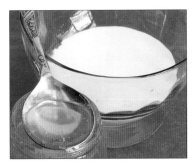 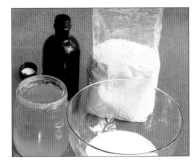

**1** To make the cleanser, mix the rose-water with the cream and stir well; make it up in small quantities and keep it in an airtight container in the fridge for up to a week.

**2** To make the face mask mix the ingredients together, including the oatmeal only if you wish to use the mixture as an exfoliating scrub. Stir well.

# ROSE AND CHAMOMILE FACIAL STEAM

*Hot-water facials open the skin's pores, creating a sense of relaxation. Fill a bowl that is just wider than your face with hot water and add 3 drops of chamomile essential oil. Cover your head with a towel and drape it over the bowl. Five minutes is usually sufficient time, but if possible relax in a darkened, quiet room for 15 minutes more before applying one of the following toning lotions.*

**Toning lotion for dry skin**
- 75 ml/5 tbsp triple-distilled rose-water
- 30 ml/2 tbsp orange-flower water

**Toning lotion for oily skin**
- 90 ml/6 tbsp triple-distilled rose-water
- 30 ml/2 tbsp witch-hazel

Combine the ingredients in a clean bottle and keep cool.

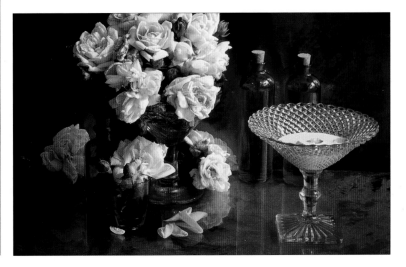

# PAPAYA FACE PACK

*Papaya fruit contains a powerful enzyme that digests dead skin. When combined with soothing aloe vera juice and green clay (a very fine clay) it becomes a gentle but effective face pack.*

- 4 medium-sized papayas
- blender or food processor
- 7.5 ml/1½ tsp aloe vera juice
- 60 ml/4 tbsp green clay
- (available from specialist suppliers)
- small glass jar, with rubber seal

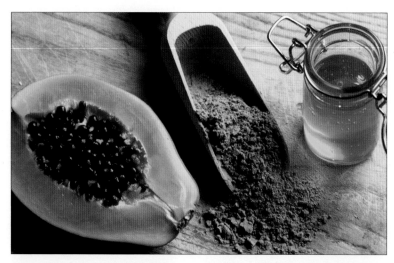

**1** Peel the papayas and blend until smooth. Add the aloe vera juice and blend again. Pour the mixture into a small bowl and slowly stir in the clay to form a smooth paste.

**2** Spoon the mix into the glass jar and either use immediately or put the lid on and use within 5 days. Store in the fridge.

**3** To use the face pack, spread the paste over your face and leave for 20 minutes before rinsing with water.

*W*arning: Test the face pack for sensitivity on a small area of your skin before using.

# GENTLE OATMEAL MASK

*This recipe is sufficient for one treatment, which must be applied immediately.*

- 15 ml/1 tbsp runny honey
- 1 egg yolk
- small bowl
- spoon
- up to 60 ml/4tbsp fine oatmeal

**1** Mix runny honey and egg yolk together in a small bowl, then slowly stir in enough oatmeal to make a soft paste.

**2** Smooth the mask on to the skin of the face and neck and leave for 15 minutes. Rinse off with lukewarm water and pat your skin dry.

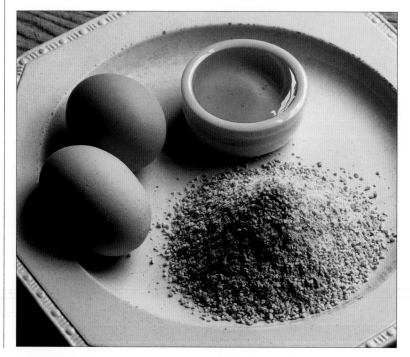

# CHAMOMILE AND HONEY MASK

*Leave the mixture on your skin for at least 10 minutes,*
*then rinse off with warm water.*

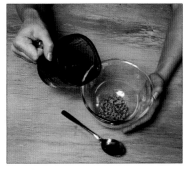

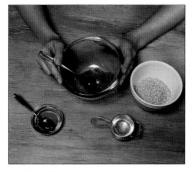

**1** Place the chamomile flowers in a heatproof bowl and pour over the boiling water. Leave to stand for 30 minutes. Strain the infusion and discard the chamomile.

**2** Mix 45 ml/3 tbsp of the liquid with the bran and honey and rub this all over your face. Leave for 15 minutes before rinsing with lukewarm water.

- 15 ml/1 tbsp dried chamomile flowers
- mixing bowl
- 175 ml/6 fl oz/¾ cup boiling water

- strainer
- 30 ml/2 tbsp bran
- 5 ml/1 tsp clear honey, warmed
- spoon

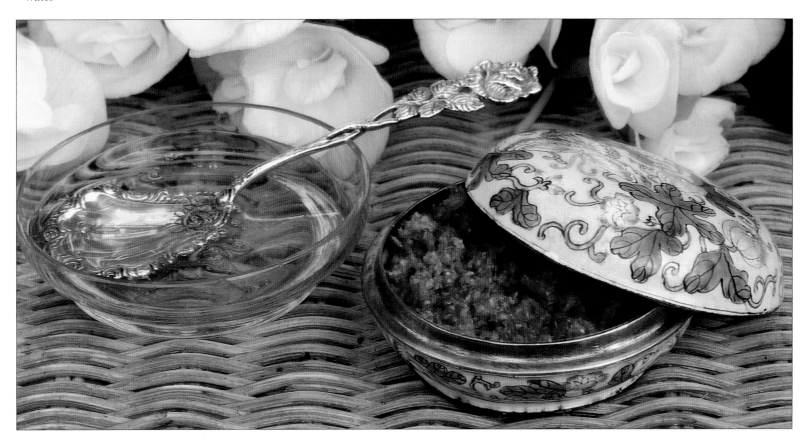

# GENTLE FACE SCRUB

*Treatment with this luxurious face scrub will cleanse your skin, leaving it silky smooth. The rose petals can be powdered in a pestle and mortar or in an electric coffee grinder. The recipe makes enough for ten treatments.*

- 45 ml/3 tbsp ground almonds (without skin)
- 45 ml/3 tbsp medium oatmeal
- 45 ml/3 tbsp powdered milk

- 30 ml/2 tbsp powdered rose petals
- glass jar, with lid
- almond oil

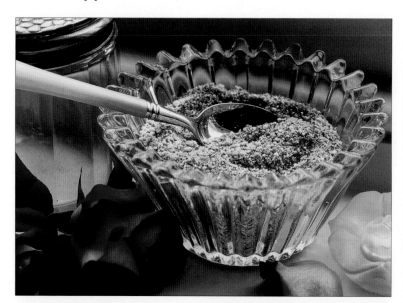

**1** Mix together the ground almonds, oatmeal, powdered milk and powdered rose petals and store the mixture in a sealed jar in the fridge.

**2** Immediately before using, mix enough for one application with some almond oil to make a soft paste. Lightly rub the paste into the skin: use a circular motion and avoid the area around the eyes. Rinse off with warm water and pat your face dry.

# ORANGE AND OATMEAL WASHING GRAINS

*For those who prefer to wash their face rather than use cleanser, this excellent once-a-week treatment exfoliates the skin, leaving it soft and glowing.*

- 30 ml/2 tbsp fine oatmeal
- 15 ml/1 tbsp powdered

- orange peel
- lidded bowl or jar

**1** Mix the oatmeal with ground orange peel and store in a lidded bowl or jar in the bathroom.

**2** To use, place a teaspoonful of the grains in the palm of one hand, mix to a paste with water and rub gently into the skin. Rinse off with warm water and pat your face dry.

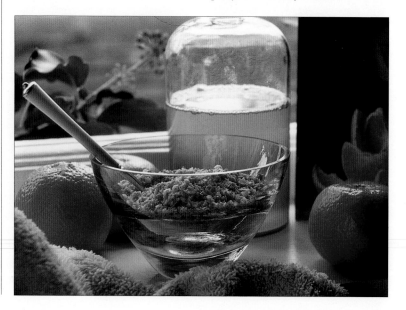

# CITRUS BODY SCRUB

*The slightly gritty texture of a scrub helps to remove dead skin cells and stimulates the skin's blood supply. The fresh citrus scent of this one is derived from the combination of orange peel and grapefruit oil. The recipe makes enough for five treatments.*

- 45 ml/3 tbsp freshly ground sunflower seeds
- 45 ml/3 tbsp medium oatmeal
- 45 ml/3 tbsp flaked sea salt
- 45 ml/3 tbsp finely grated orange peel
- 3 drops grapefruit essential oil
- mixing bowl
- glass jar, with lid
- almond oil

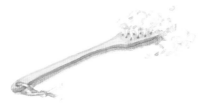

**2** Rub the paste over the body, taking care to include areas of hard, dry skin such as elbows, knees and ankles. Remove the residue before bathing or showering. Store the remainder in the fridge.

**1** Thoroughly mix all the ingredients, except for the almond oil, together in a bowl, then store them in the jar. Blend one fifth of the mixture with sufficient almond oil to make a paste.

# LUXURIOUS AFTER-BATH SCRUB

*Dry your skin thoroughly before rubbing this mixture into dry areas, and leave to dry. Rub it off using a soft flannel while standing in the bath.*

- 30 ml/2 tbsp powdered orange peel
- 45 ml/3 tbsp ground almonds
- 30 ml/2 tbsp oatmeal
- 15 ml/1 tbsp red rose petals
- mixing bowl and spoon
- 90 ml/6 tbsp almond oil
- 5 drops flower oil (jasmine, rose, neroli or lavender)
- 5 drops wood oil (sandalwood, rosewood or cedar)
- glass jar or bottle, with lid

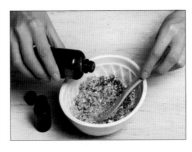

Mix all the dry ingredients together. Add the almond oil, a little at a time, blending the mixture to a crumbly paste. Stir in the the essential oils of your choice and transfer to a glass jar or bottle. Use within 2 weeks.

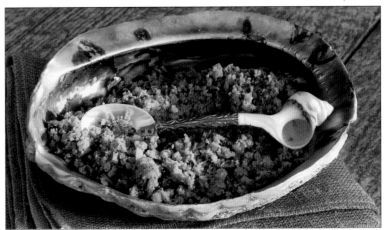

# HERBAL WASH BALLS

❧

*Perfumed soap balls make wonderful gifts, especially when they are gathered up in pretty pouches. In addition to lavender, soap balls can be fragranced with other essential oils, such as pure rose or neroli.*

- 1 large bar unscented soap
- grater
- measuring jug
- double boiler
- spoon
- pestle and mortar
- lavender essential oil
- organza, 30 cm/ 12 in square
- scissors
- taffeta ribbon

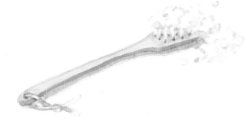

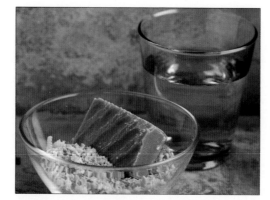

**1** Finely grate the bar of unscented soap. Measure out some water: you will need 1 part water to 2 parts soap.

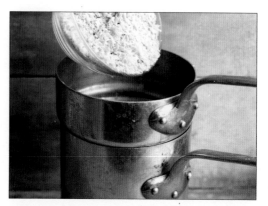

**2** Put the water and soap into a double boiler and gently heat, stirring continuously, until you have a thick paste.

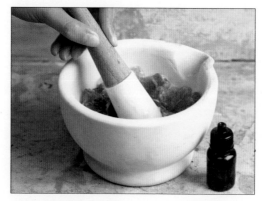

**3** Transfer the paste to a mortar and add 12 drops of lavender oil to each 150 g/5 oz of the original soap. Pound with the pestle and mix thoroughly.

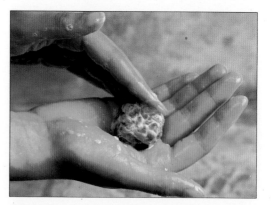

**4** Wet your hands and roll a small amount of the mixture into a ball. Repeat with the rest of the soap and leave to set. When dry, the balls can be packaged in a square of organza prettily tied with a taffeta ribbon.

*To* make the balls more decorative, you can press fresh rose petals or lavender flowers into the surface while the mixture is still moist and soft.

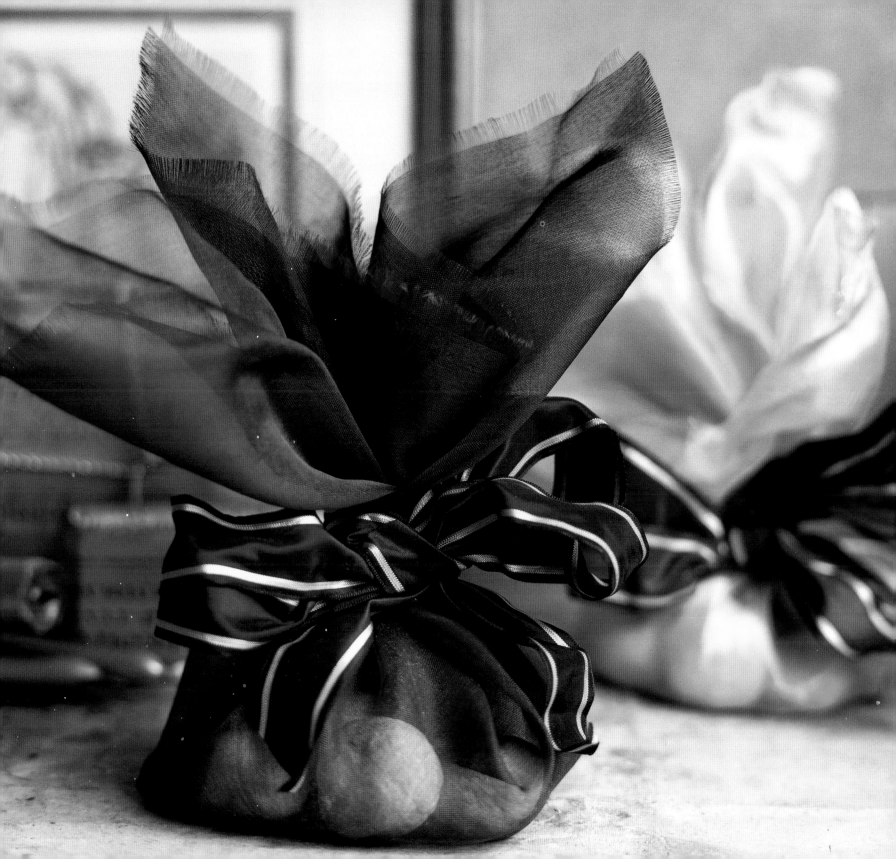

# Olive Oil and Lavender Soap

*Enrich a block of green Marseilles olive-oil soap with other oils and finely ground almonds and then scent it with lavender, to make pretty guest soaps. In the process, the olive oils partially settle out, to create an interesting marbled effect.*

- 175 g/6 oz olive oil soap
- grater
- double boiler
- 25 ml/1½ tbsp coconut oil
- 25 ml/1½ tbsp almond oil
- 30 ml/2 tbsp ground almonds
- 10 drops lavender essential oil
- spoon
- heart-shaped moulds, oiled

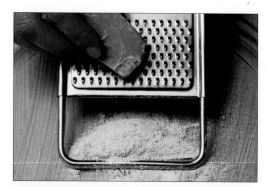

**1** Grate the soap. Place the grated soap in a double boiler and leave to soften over heat. Add all the other ingredients.

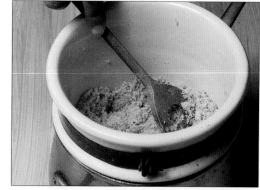

**2** Stir until all the ingredients are evenly mixed and begin to hold together.

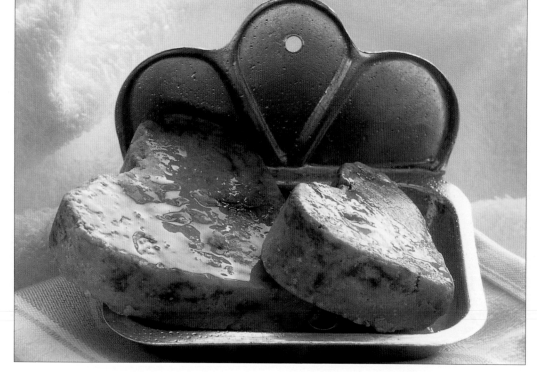

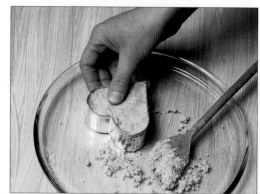

**3** Press the mixture into the oiled moulds and leave to set overnight. Unmould the soaps ready for use.

# MARIGOLD AND SUNFLOWER SOAP

*This sunny soap has been made from unscented vegetable glycerine soap, with added oils, ground sunflower seeds and marigold petals; it is scented with bergamot oil, which gives it a light citrus fragrance. Make as for Olive Oil and Lavender Soap. These soaps are moulded into heart shapes, but you could simply roll them into balls.*

- 175 g/6 oz vegetable glycerine soap
- grater
- double boiler
- 25 ml/1½ tbsp coconut oil
- 25 ml/1½ tbsp almond oil
- 30 ml/2 tbsp finely ground sunflower seeds
- 15 ml/1 tbsp dried marigold petals
- 10 drops bergamot essential oil
- spoon
- heart-shaped moulds, oiled

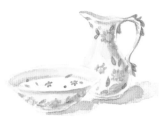

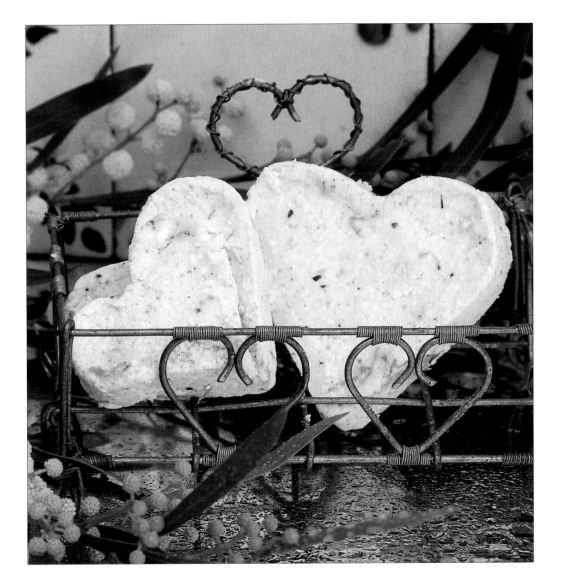

When remodelling soap at home, it is essential to use only simple vegetable, glycerine or olive-oil soaps as other types would be difficult to work with. Both soaps shown here include almond and coconut oils for richness and an essential oil for scent. Ground nuts or seeds are included to give a gentle exfoliating action.

# PARSLEY HAIR TONIC

*Parsley helps to stimulate the circulation in the scalp, which aids hair growth and leaves your hair looking healthy and glossy.*

- 1 large handful parsley sprigs
- blender or food processor

- 30 ml/2 tbsp water

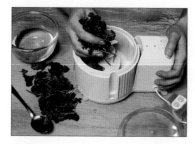

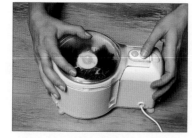

**1** Place the parsley in a blender or food processor with the water.

**2** Process until the parsley is ground to a smooth, green purée. Apply the lotion to your scalp, then wrap a warm towel around your head. Leave for about an hour before washing your hair as usual.

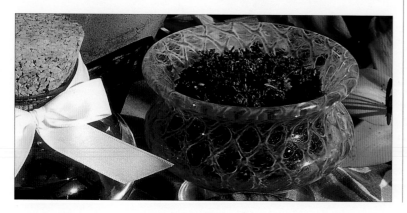

# ROSEMARY HAIR TONIC

*Rosemary can be used as a substitute for mildly medicated shampoos. It is also effective in controlling greasy hair and enhances the shine and natural colour, especially of dark hair. Use this tonic as a final rinse after shampooing, catching it in a bowl and pouring it repeatedly through the hair.*

- 250 ml/8 fl oz/1 cup fresh rosemary tips
- 1.2 litres/2 pints/5 cups bottled water

- saucepan
- strainer
- bottle

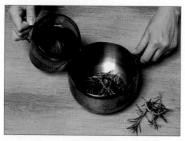

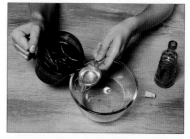

**1** Place all the rosemary and water in a saucepan and bring to the boil. Simmer for approximately 20 minutes, then allow to cool in the pan.

**2** Strain the liquid and store it in a clean bottle. Apply it to your hair after shampooing normally.

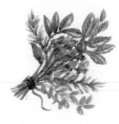

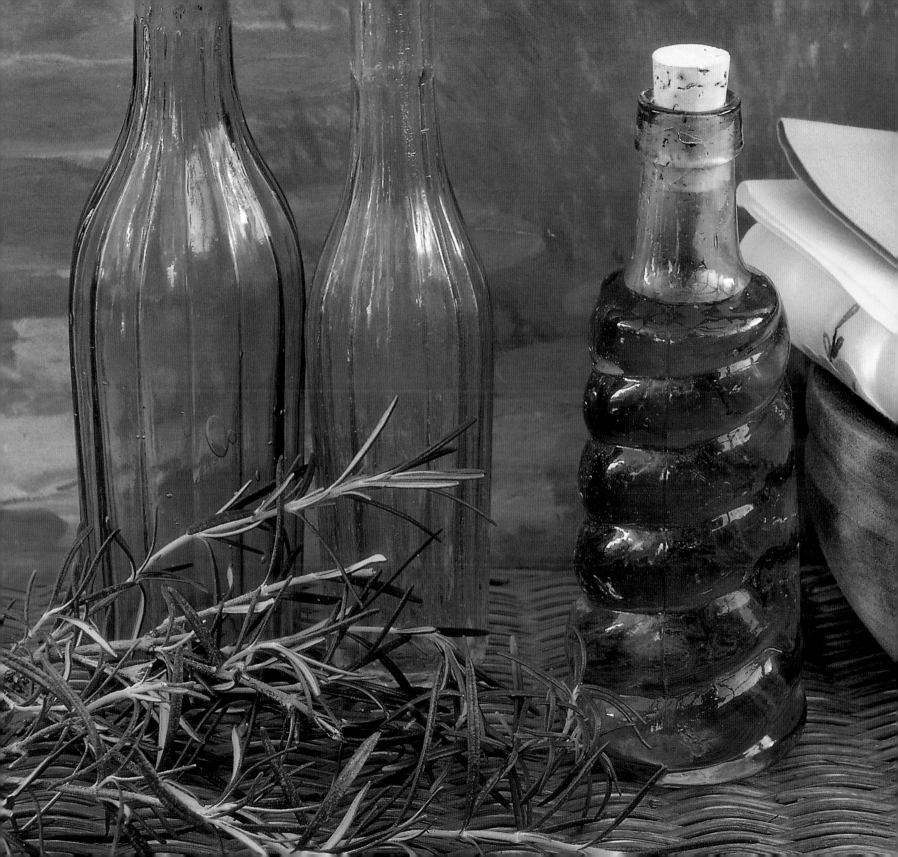

# LEMON VERBENA HAIR RINSE

*This rinse will fragrance your hair wonderfully as well as stimulating the pores and circulation of the scalp.*
*Lemon verbena is easy to grow in the garden.*

- 250 ml/8 fl oz/
  1 cup boiling water
- 1 handful lemon
  verbena leaves

- bowl
- jug
- strainer

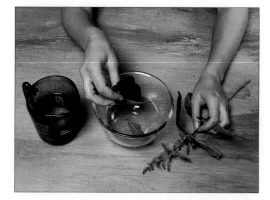

**1** Pour the boiling water over the lemon
verbena leaves and infuse for at least an hour.

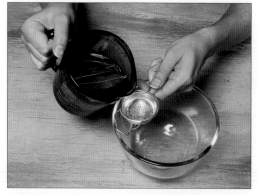

**2** Strain the liquid and discard the leaves. Pour
the rinse over your hair after conditioning.

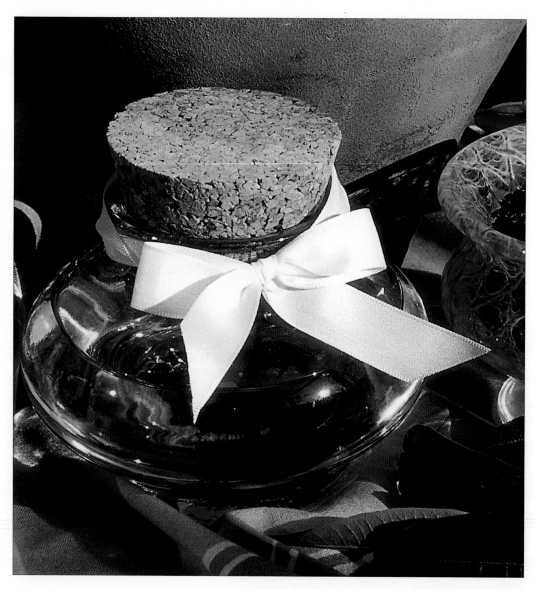

# CHAMOMILE CONDITIONING RINSE

*Chamomile flowers will not affect the colour of medium to dark hair, but they will help to brighten naturally fair hair.*
*Their pleasant fragrance is combined here with scented geranium.*

- 125 ml/4 fl oz/
  ½ cup chamomile
  flowers
- 600 ml/1 pint/
  2½ cups water
- saucepan
- strainer
- bowl
- 1 handful scented
  geranium leaves
- bottle

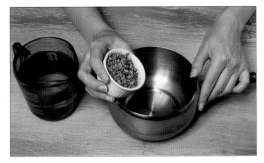

Place the flowers and water in a saucepan and bring to the boil. Simmer for 15 minutes.

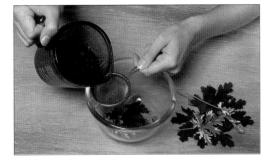

**2** Strain the still hot liquid over the scented geranium leaves and leave them to soak for 30–40 minutes. Strain into a bottle. Use the rinse after shampooing normally.

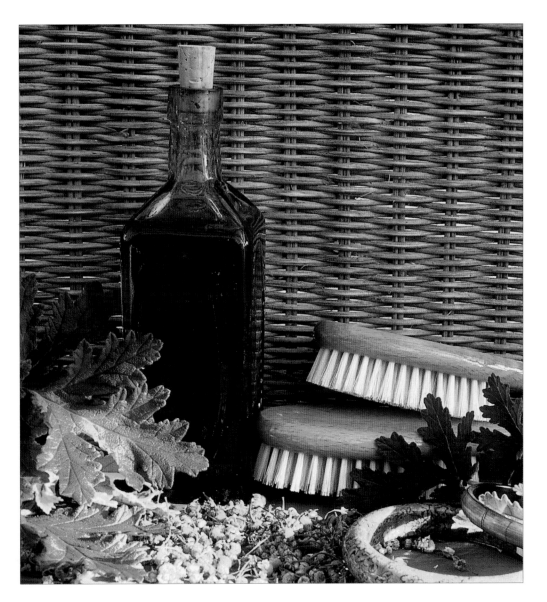

# CIDER VINEGAR HAIR RINSE

*This traditional country beauty treatment invigorates the scalp and gives hair a deep shine.*
*This preparation makes enough for one treatment.*

- 250 ml/8 fl oz/
  1 cup cider vinegar
- 1 litre/1¾ pints/
  4 cups warm water

Mix the cider with the warm water and use as a final rinse for the hair. Towel dry, gently comb through and leave to dry naturally.

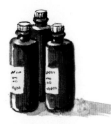

## VARIATIONS

Different rinses using natural ingredients can be made at home to correct a variety of hair problems. To make these, place 30 ml/2 tbsp of the appropriate fresh herb in a china or glass bowl, add 600 ml/1 pint/2½ cups boiling water, cover and leave for 3 hours. The longer the herbs steep, the stronger the infusion will be. Strain before using. Fresh herbs are better, but if you only have access to dried herbs, halve the amount.

Use the following herbs for specific problems:
- Southernwood to combat grease.
- Nettles to stimulate hair growth.
- Rosemary to prevent static.
- Lavender to soothe a tight scalp.

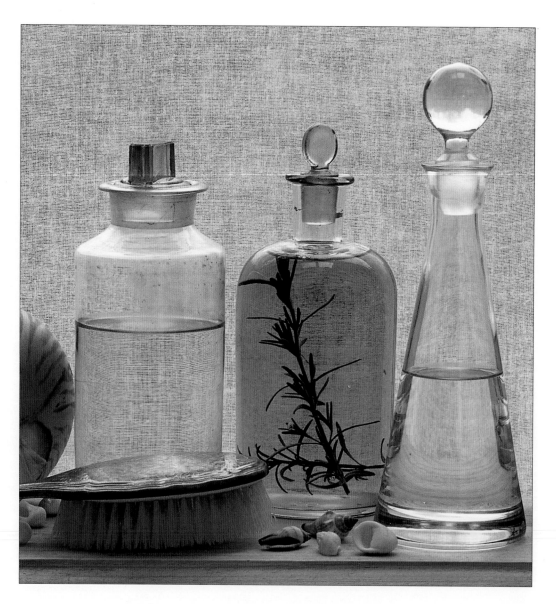

# HAIR RESCUER

*To improve the condition of dry and damaged hair, apply this mixture after shampooing and comb through. Leave for 5 minutes before rinsing.*

- 30 ml/2 tbsp olive oil
- 30 ml/2 tbsp light sesame oil
- 2 eggs
- 30 ml/2 tbsp coconut milk

- 30 ml/2 tbsp runny honey
- 5 ml/1 tsp coconut oil
- blender or food processor
- bottle

**1** Process all the ingredients until smooth.

**2** Transfer to a bottle. Keep in the fridge and use within 3 days.

# WARM-OIL TREATMENT

*Applied once a month, this treatment should improve the texture of your hair and condition your scalp.*

- 90 ml/6 tbsp coconut oil
- 3 drops rosemary essential oil
- 2 drops tea tree essential oil

- 2 drops lavender essential oil
- dark-coloured glass bottle with stopper

**1** Pour all the ingredients into the bottle and shake gently to mix. Use the oil sparingly on dry hair; the head should not be soaked.

**2** Massage the oil in, then cover your head with a hot towel for 20 minutes. Shampoo as normal.

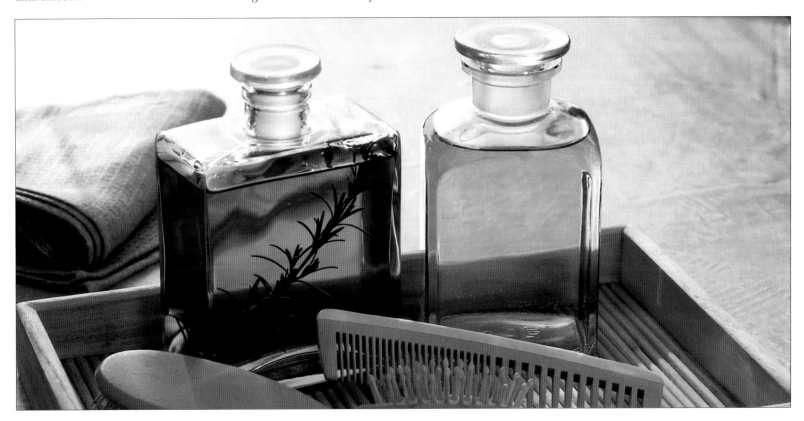

# MOISTURIZING AND MASSAGE

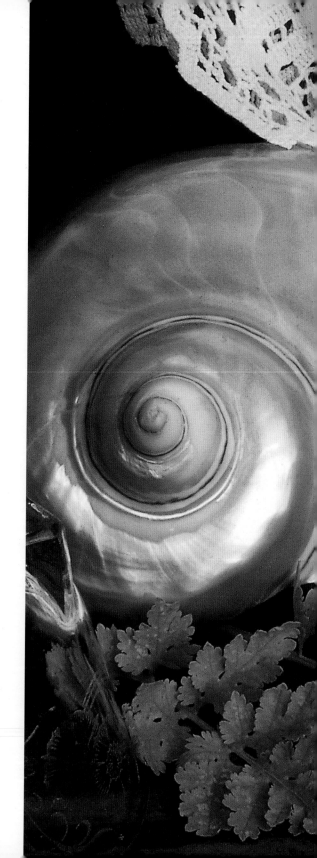

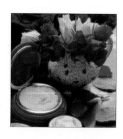

*O*nce your skin has been thoroughly cleansed, it is ready to be toned and moisturized. The recipes on the following pages cater for a variety of skin types and include specific treatments for face, hands, nails and feet as well as creams and oils that will nourish and invigorate the skin generally. Lotions and moisturizers are easy and satisfying to make from the finest natural ingredients, and

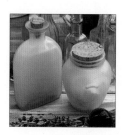

you can add delicious scents using your favourite essential oils. A range of scented massage oils is also included here, to help restore tired, tense muscles, reduce stress and relax the whole body.

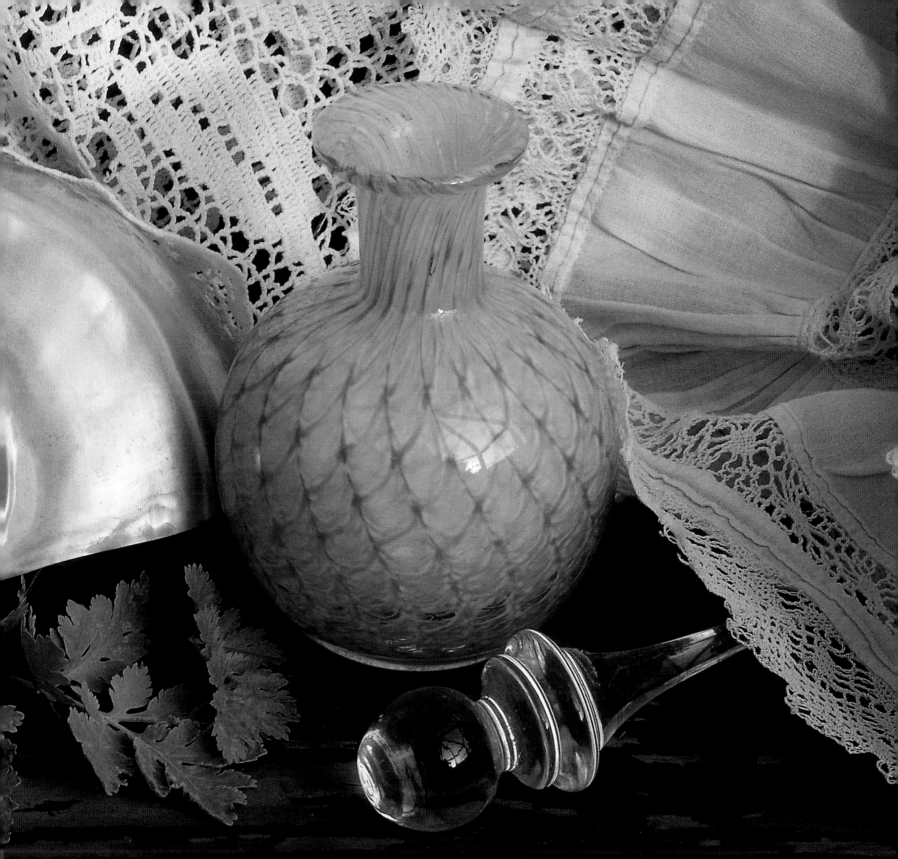

# $\mathcal{E}$LDERFLOWER SKIN FRESHENER

*Skin fresheners and tonics can be made up according to skin type, using natural ingredients with known beneficial effects. Here, the recipe is modified by including cider vinegar for normal skin, witch-hazel for slightly oily skin, or vodka for very oily skin and open pores. Use the freshener by pouring a small amount on to a dampened piece of cotton wool.*

- 10 elderflower heads
- heatproof mixing bowl
- 300 ml/½ pint/ 1¼ cups bottled water

- clean dish towel
- 15 ml/1 tbsp cider vinegar, witch-hazel or vodka
- strainer
- glass jar, with lid

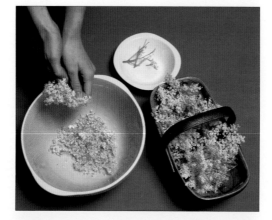

**1** Wash the elderflower heads briefly and make sure they are free of insects. Strip the flowerheads from the stems and place them in the heatproof bowl.

## VARIATIONS

Different formulations of skin tonic can be used to soothe or stimulate skin. Prepare them by pouring the ingredients into a glass bottle and shaking them well to mix. Make flower infusions as for Elderflower Skin Freshener.

ORANGE-FLOWER SKIN TONIC (normal skin)
- 75 ml/5 tbsp orange-flower water
- 25 ml/1½ tbsp rose-water

CORNFLOWER SKIN TONIC (normal skin)
- 75 ml/5 tbsp cornflower infusion
- 25 ml/1½ tbsp rose-water

LAVENDER SKIN TONIC (oily skin)
- 75 ml/5 tbsp lavender infusion
- 25 ml/1½ tbsp witch-hazel

LINDEN SKIN TONIC (mature skin)
- 90 ml/6 tbsp lime-flower infusion
- 10 ml/2 tsp rose-water

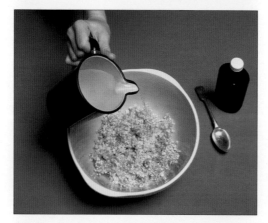

**2** Bring the water to the boil in a saucepan and pour it over the flowerheads. Cover with a dish towel and leave for 20 minutes. Add the cider vinegar, witch-hazel or vodka, cover and leave overnight to infuse.

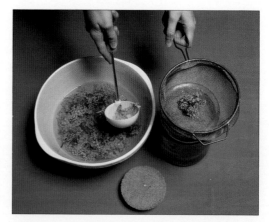

**3** Strain the liquid into the jar. Cover and leave to cool. Store in the fridge.

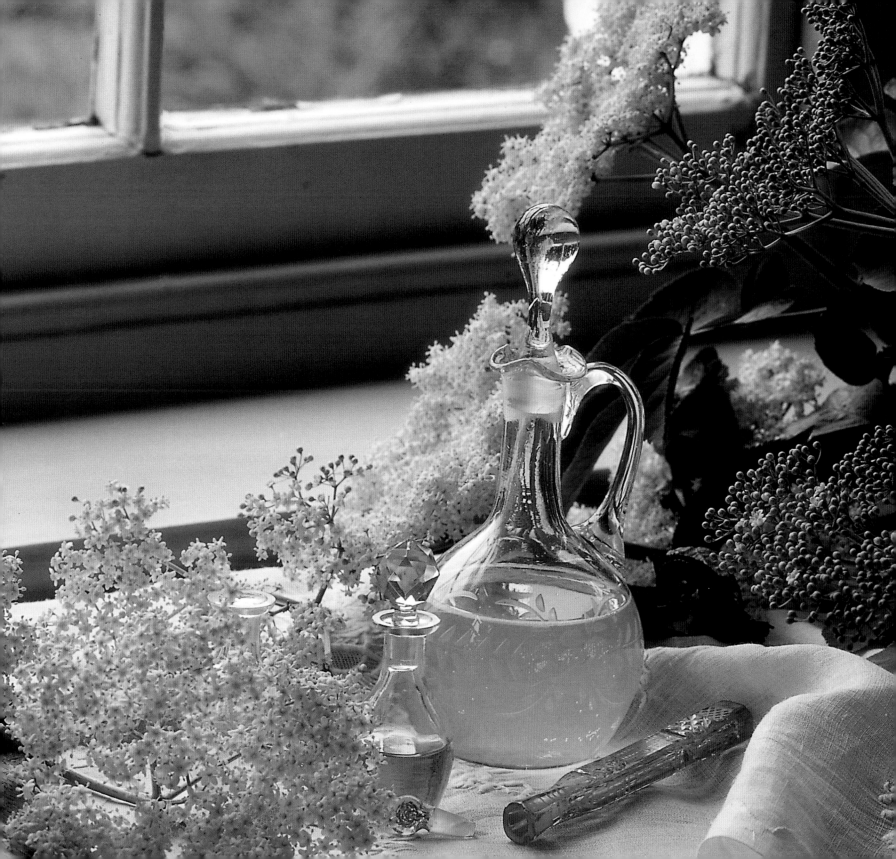

# TANSY SKIN FRESHENER

*Tansy leaves are fairly strong smelling and this tonic will invigorate your skin first thing in the morning.*

- 1 large handful tansy leaves
- 150 ml/¼ pint/ ⅔ cup water
- 150 ml/¼ pint/

- ⅔ cup milk
- saucepan
- strainer
- bottle

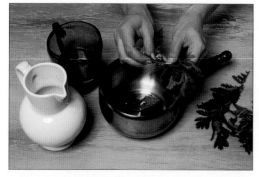

**1** Place all the ingredients in a small pan and bring to the boil. Simmer for 15 minutes, then remove from the heat and allow to cool.

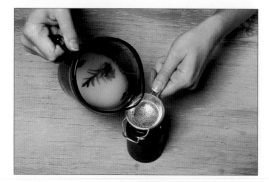

**2** Strain the liquid into a bottle. Keep the tonic in the fridge, and apply cold to the skin.

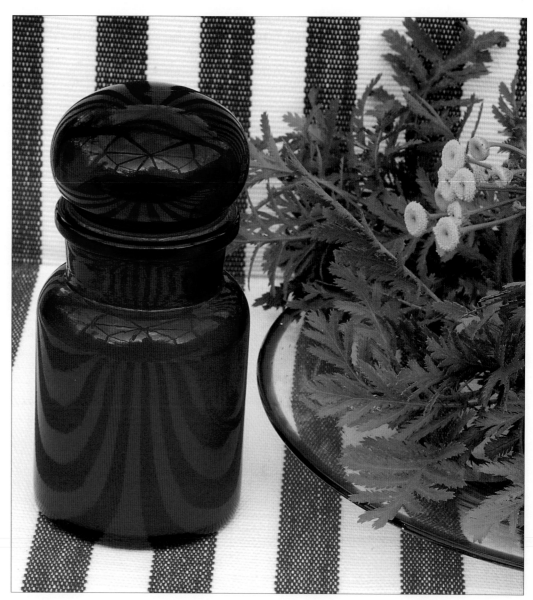

# FEVERFEW COMPLEXION MILK

*Feverfew milk is excellent for moisturizing dry skin, helping to fade blemishes and discourage blackheads.*
*Feverfew is easy to grow in the garden and self-seeds prodigiously.*

- 1 large handful feverfew leaves
- 300 ml/½ pint/ 1¼ cups milk

- saucepan
- strainer
- bottle

**1** Place the feverfew leaves and milk in a small saucepan, bring to the boil, then reduce the heat and simmer for 20 minutes.

**2** Remove from the heat and allow the mixture to cool in the pan. Strain into a bottle and store in the fridge.

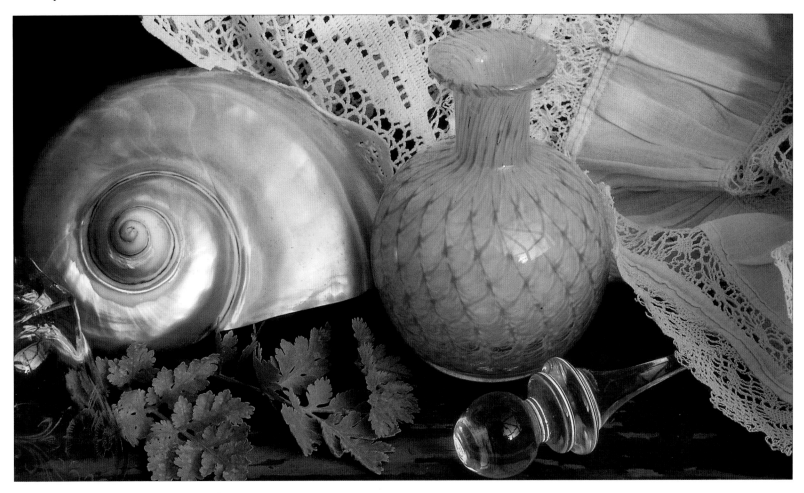

# LAVENDER MOISTURIZER

*Lavender is the ideal essential oil to use in a face cream as it not only smells wonderful but also helps to heal skin blemishes.*

- 20 ml/4 tsp beeswax granules
- 20 g/¾ oz cocoa butter
- 75 ml/5 tbsp almond oil
- 10 ml/2 tsp borax
- 175 ml/6 fl oz/¾ cup lavender water

- mixing bowl
- 2 saucepans
- spoon
- 8 drops lavender essential oil
- decorative glass jars, with lids

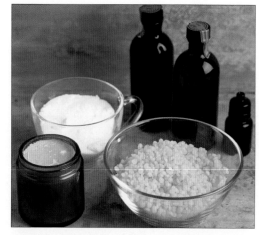

**1** Measure out the beeswax granules, cocoa butter, almond oil, borax and lavender water to the amounts required.

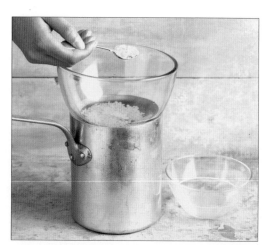

**2** Put the beeswax, cocoa butter and almond oil in a bowl set over a saucepan of simmering water and melt, stirring constantly. In a separate saucepan, dissolve the borax in the lavender water by gently warming it. Add the lavender water and borax to the melted mixture in the bowl, stirring constantly.

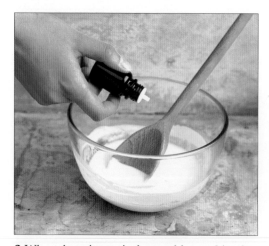

**3** When the mixture is thoroughly combined, remove it from the heat and allow to cool. While still tepid, mix in the lavender oil.

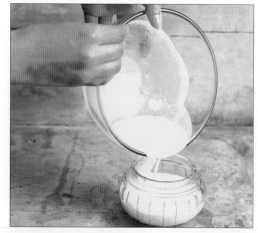

**4** Pour the moisturizer into glass jars. Store in the fridge for up to 3 weeks.

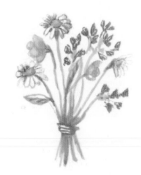

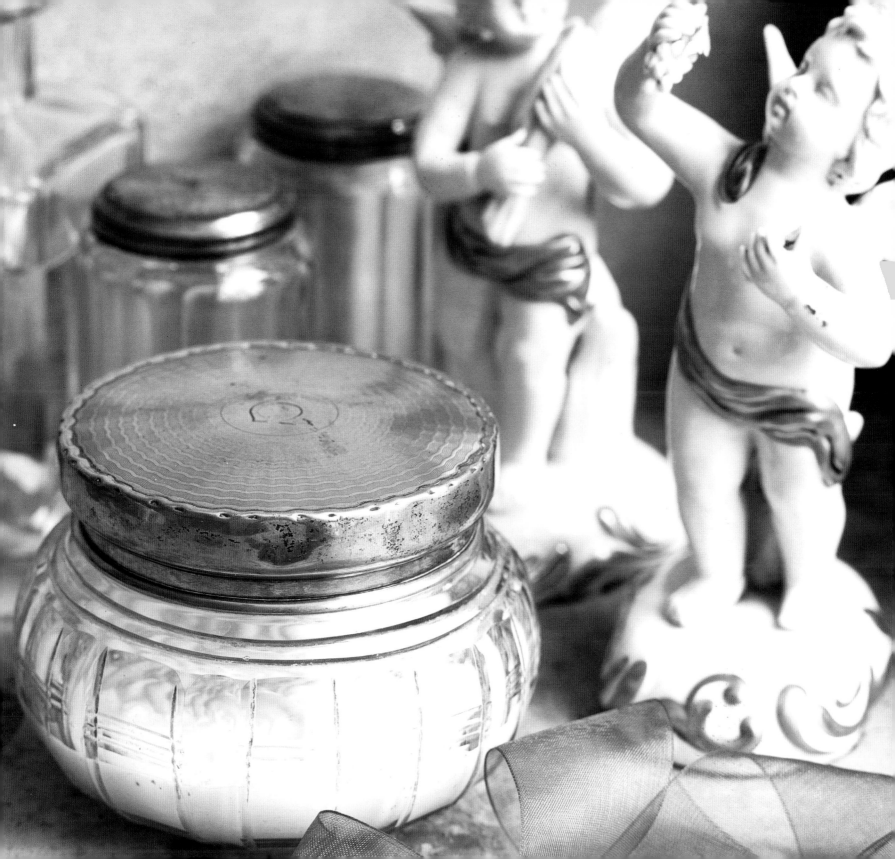

# TRADITIONAL COLD CREAM

*This basic cream can be used to cleanse and soothe skin.*

- 50 g/2 oz white beeswax
- double boiler
- 115 g/4 oz almond oil
- spoon

- 2.5ml/½ tsp borax
- 50 ml/2 fl oz/ ¼ cup rose-water
- whisk
- glass or china pots

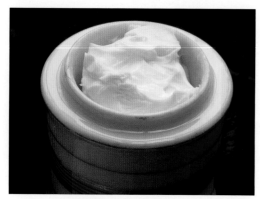

## UNSCENTED MOISTURE CREAM

Excellent for applying before going outdoors, this simple cream can be used by both men and women. Melt the waxes with the oil in a double boiler over a gentle heat, and stir. Remove from the heat, then pour the cream into a pot to set.

- 30 ml/2 tbsp carnauba wax
- 15 ml/1 tbsp white beeswax
- 120 ml/4 fl oz/

½ cup almond oil
- double boiler
- spoon
- glass or china pot

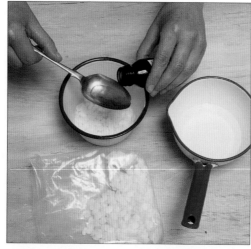

**1** Place the beeswax in a double boiler and add the almond oil. Melt the wax over a gentle heat, stirring continuously to combine the ingredients.

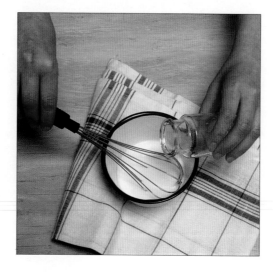

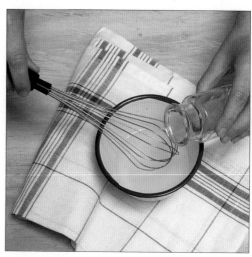

**2** Remove from the heat and dissolve the borax in the rose-water. Slowly pour this into the melted wax and oil, whisking continuously.

**3** The mixture will quickly turn milky and thicken. Continue whisking as it cools. When it reaches a thick, pouring consistency, pour it into glass or china pots.

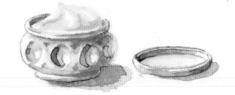

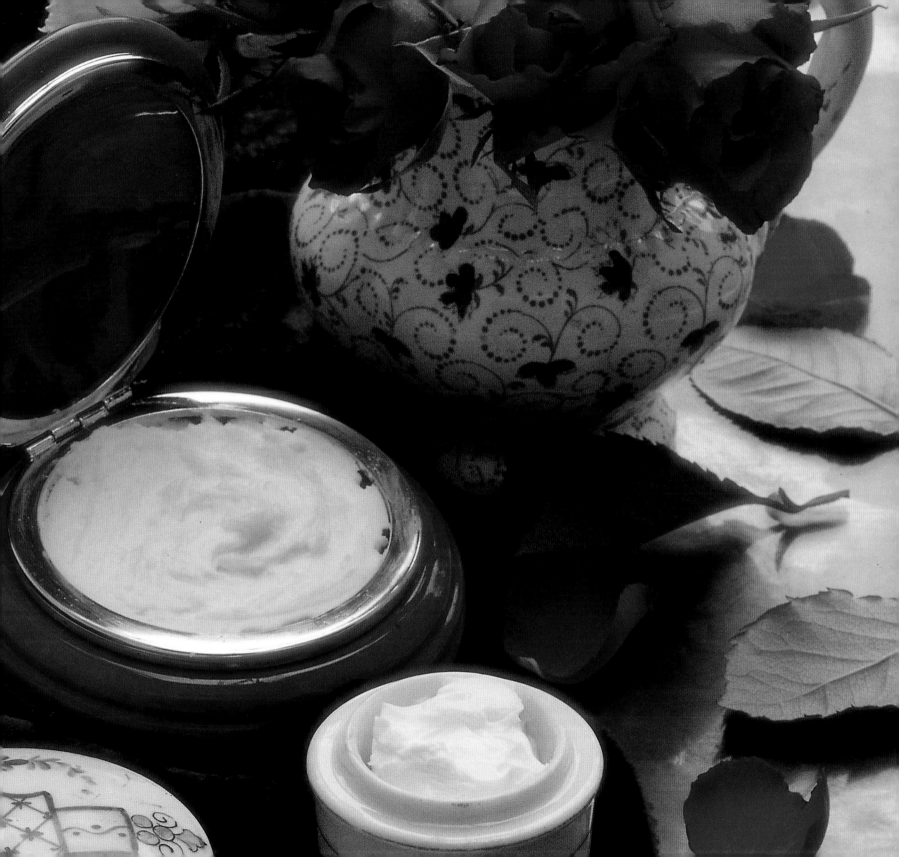

# ROSE HAND CREAM

*Applied regularly, this fragrant hand cream, which is rich in nourishing oils and waxes, keeps skin in good condition.*

- 50 ml/2 fl oz/¼ cup rose-water
- 45 ml/3 tbsp witch-hazel
- 2.5 ml/½ tsp glycerine
- 1.5 ml/¼ tsp borax
- saucepan
- 30 ml/2 tbsp

- emulsifying wax or white beeswax
- double boiler
- 5 ml/1 tsp lanolin
- 30 ml/2 tbsp almond oil
- 2 drops rose essential oil
- glass or china pots

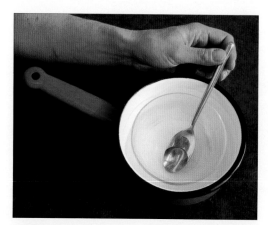

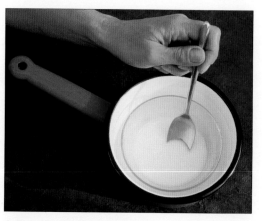

**1** Place the rose-water, witch-hazel, glycerine and borax in a saucepan and gently heat until the borax has dissolved. In a double boiler, melt the wax, lanolin and almond oil over a gentle heat.

**2** Slowly add the rose-water mixture to the oil mixture, stirring constantly. It will quickly turn milky and thicken. Remove from the heat and continue to stir while it cools. When cool, add the rose essential oil. Pour the cream into glass or china pots and store in a cool place.

## ROSE NAIL OIL

Massaging the base of your nails every day with this oil will encourage healthy growth. The oil can also be used as part of a manicure: soak the nails for at least 10 minutes after you have thoroughly cleaned them. To make the oil, simply mix the ingredients together and store in a dark coloured bottle.

- 50 ml/2 fl oz/¼ cup almond oil
- 10 ml/2 tsp apricot kernel oil

- 5 drops geranium essential oil
- 2 drops rose essential oil

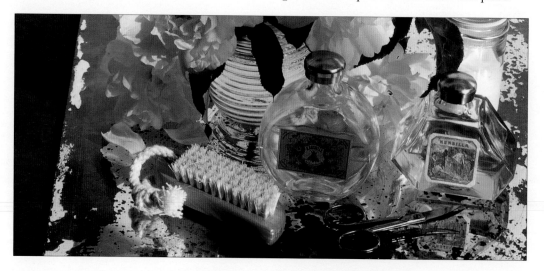

# WINTER HAND CREAM

*This very nourishing cream includes patchouli oil, which is a good healer of cracked and chapped skin.*
*Consequently it is an ideal ointment for hands roughened and sore from gardening activities.*

- grater
- 75 g/3 oz unscented, hard white soap
- bowl
- 90 ml/6 tbsp boiling water
- spoon
- 115 g/4 oz beeswax
- 45 ml/3 tbsp glycerine
- 150 ml/¼ pint/ ⅔ cup almond oil
- 45 ml/3 tbsp rose-water
- double boiler
- whisk
- 25 drops patchouli oil
- glass or china pots or jars

## HEALING HAND CREAM

Perfect for using on little cuts and scratches, this is also a real barrier cream against moisture. Place the petroleum jelly, paraffin wax and lanolin in a double boiler and melt slowly over a gentle heat, stirring continuously. When melted, remove from the heat and continue stirring as the mixture cools and thickens. Stir in the essential oil and store in a china or dark glass container.

- 90 ml/6 tbsp white petroleum jelly
- 2.5 ml/½ tsp paraffin wax
- 1.5 ml/¼ tsp anhydrous lanolin
- double boiler
- spoon
- 10 drops essential oil (lemon, tea tree or lavender)
- china or dark glass container

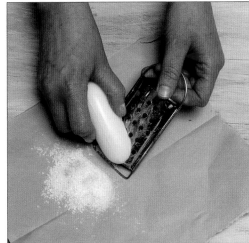

**1** Grate the soap and place it in a bowl. Pour the boiling water over the grated soap and stir until smooth.

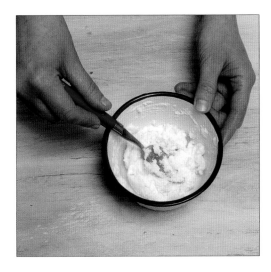

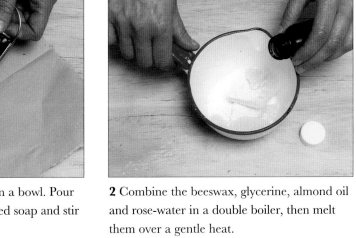

**2** Combine the beeswax, glycerine, almond oil and rose-water in a double boiler, then melt them over a gentle heat.

**3** Remove from the heat and gradually whisk in the soap mixture. Continue whisking as the mixture cools and thickens. Stir in the patchouli oil and pour into glass or china pots or jars.

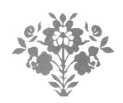

# MINT FOOTBATH AND MASSAGE OIL

*Soaking tired feet at the end of the day will revitalize your entire body, and rubbing mint oil into your feet before going to bed will smooth and soften them. The refreshing scent of the mint essential oil enhances the whole soothing treatment.*

**Mint footbath**
- 12 large sprigs mint
- blender or food processor
- 120 ml/4 fl oz/½ cup cold water
- large bowl

- 2.4 litres/4 pints/10 cups boiling water

**Massage oil**
- 15 ml/1 tbsp almond oil
- 1 drop mint essential oil

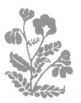

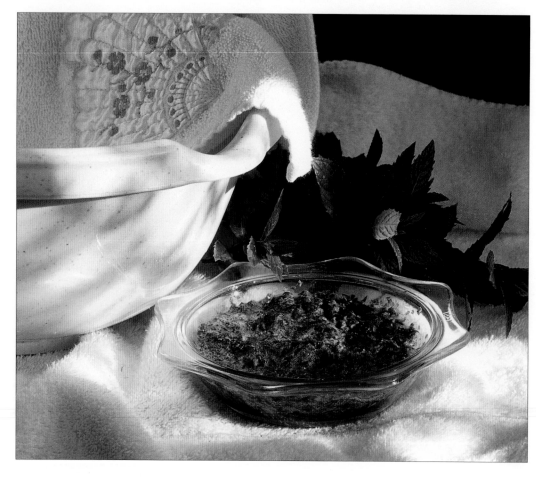

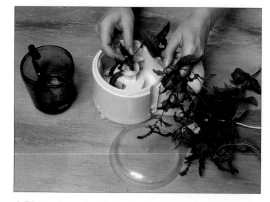

**1** Place the mint in a food processor and add the cold water. Process to a green purée. Pour the purée into a large bowl and add the boiling water. Allow to cool to a bearable temperature, then soak both feet at once until the water is no longer comforting.

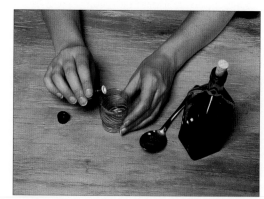

**2** Gently dry your feet with a soft towel. Mix the almond oil and the mint essential oil together and rub this well into both feet.

# TEA TREE FOOT CREAM AND BODY LOTION

*Tea tree is one of the great healing oils, with antiseptic and fungicidal properties which will protect the feet from foot complaints often acquired at the swimming pool or gym. Its fresh resinous smell makes it an ideal oil for both men and women. For ease of use, the foot cream can be kept in a pump-action plastic bottle rather than in the more usual glass or ceramic container.*

**Foot cream**
- 15 drops tea tree essential oil
- 120 ml/4 fl oz/$\frac{1}{2}$ cup unscented hand cream
- funnel
- pump-action plastic bottle

**Body lotion**
- 2.5 ml/$\frac{1}{2}$ tsp borax
- 60 ml/4 tbsp boiled water

- 7.5 ml/$\frac{1}{2}$ tbsp white beeswax
- 45 ml/3 tbsp coconut oil
- 30 ml/2 tbsp almond oil
- 15 ml/1 tbsp wheatgerm oil
- double boiler
- whisk
- 20 drops tea tree oil
- coloured glass bottle or jar

**1** For the foot cream, blend the essential oil thoroughly into the unscented hand cream and pour into the plastic bottle.

**2** For the body lotion, dissolve the borax in the water. Melt the beeswax with the coconut, almond and wheatgerm oils in a double boiler over a gentle heat.

**3** When completely melted, remove from the heat and slowly pour in the borax solution, while stirring continuously with a whisk. The lotion will begin to turn milky and thicken immediately.

**4** Continue to whisk until the mixture has cooled, then add the tea tree oil. Pour the lotion into a coloured glass bottle or jar and store in a cool place.

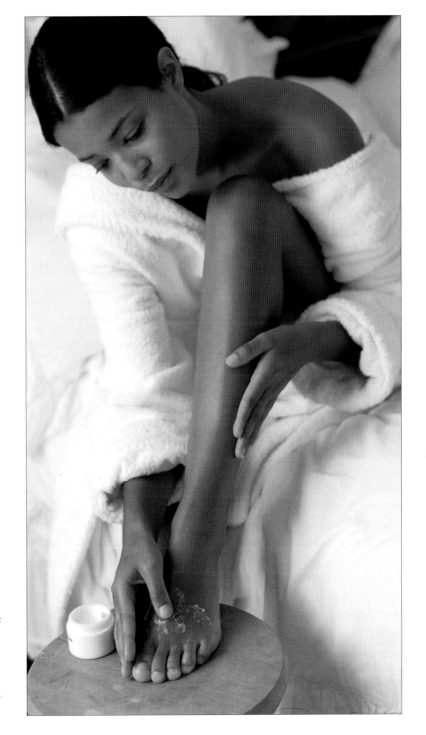

# LAVENDER BODY LOTION

*This creamy lotion is excellent for conditioning dry skin in winter, and because lavender oil is an effective treatment for burns, it can also be used to soothe sunburn.*

- 1.5 ml/¼ tsp borax
- 30 ml/2tbsp boiled water
- 5 ml/1 tsp white beeswax
- 5 ml/1 tsp lanolin
- 30 ml/2 tbsp petroleum jelly
- 25 ml/5 tsp apricot kernel oil
- 20 ml/4 tsp cold-pressed sunflower oil
- double boiler
- whisk
- 20 drops lavender oil
- glass jar or bottle

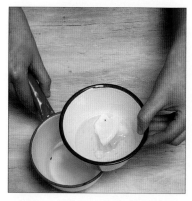

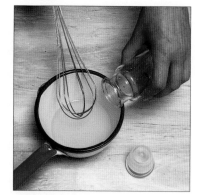

**1** Dissolve the borax in the boiled water. Melt the beeswax, lanolin and petroleum jelly with the apricot kernel oil and cold-pressed sunflower oil in a double boiler. When melted, remove from the heat and stir well to blend.

**2** Add the borax solution, whisking continuously. The lotion will turn white and thicken, but continue whisking it until cool. Stir in the lavender oil. Pour the lotion into a glass jar or bottle and store in a cool, dark place.

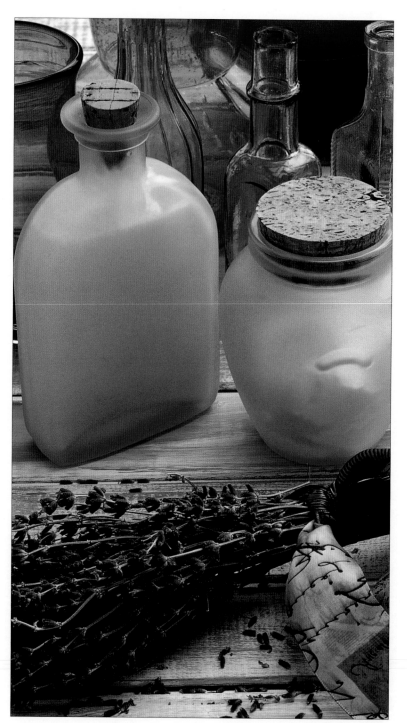

# ROSE BODY LOTION

*A fragrant lotion, reminiscent of high summer and romance.*
*Rose oil is excellent for all skin types. This frosted glass bottle*
*has been decorated with gilded rose leaves and a gold label*
*with a heart motif.*

- 175 ml/6 fl oz/¾ cup
  unscented body lotion
- 10 drops rose essential oil
- decorative, screw-topped bottle

Mix the body lotion and rose oil together thoroughly and pour into a decorative bottle.

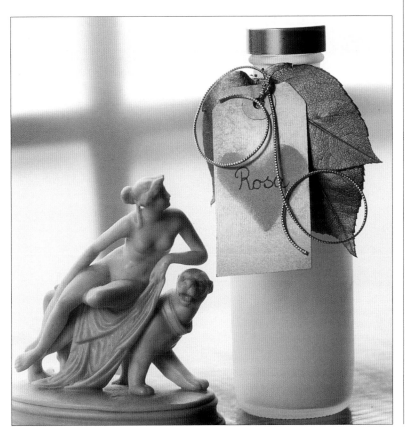

# GERANIUM BODY LOTION

*This spicily fragrant lotion is pleasantly aromatic.*
*Geranium oil is derived from a relative of the scented leaf*
*geranium and the fragrance is very like that of the crushed leaves.*
*This bottle has been decorated with a geranium leaf and*
*a gilded, heart-shaped label.*

- 175 ml/6 fl oz/¾ cup
  unscented body lotion
- 15 drops geranium essential oil
- decorative, screw-topped bottle

Mix the body lotion and geranium oil together thoroughly and pour into a decorative bottle.

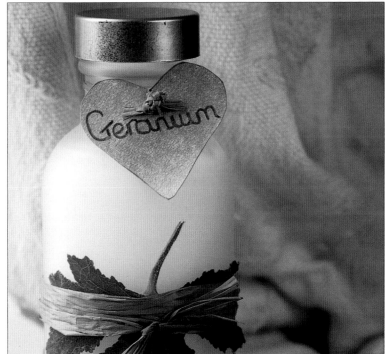

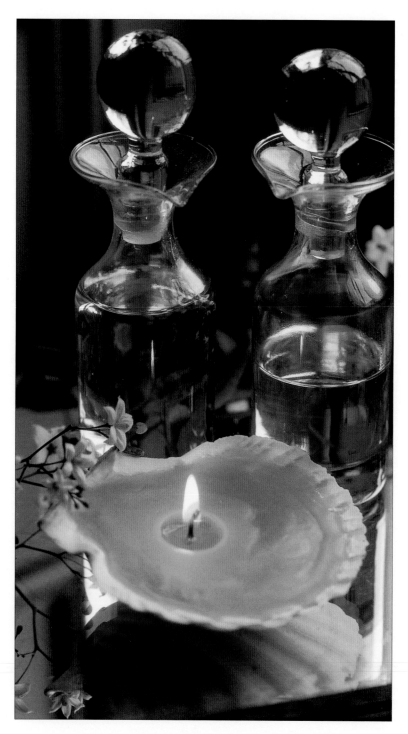

# SOOTHING
## MASS AGE OIL

*This pleasant blend of oils is ideal for soothing away stress
and nervous headaches. When a full massage is not possible,
rub a few drops of the oil behind the ears in a circular motion.
Clary sage and chamomile should be avoided during pregnancy.*

- 45 ml/3 tbsp almond oil
- 1.5 ml/¼ tsp wheatgerm oil
- 10 drops lavender essential oil
- 5 drops clary sage essential oil
- 5 drops chamomile essential oil
- glass bottle

Pour all the ingredients into a glass bottle with a stopper and gently
shake to mix. Store in a cool, dark place.

# SEDUCTIVE
## MASS AGE OIL

*Some of the essential oils are said to have aphrodisiac qualities.
Among the more sensuous are rose, jasmine, neroli and ylang-ylang.
Two types of pure rose oil, rose otto (attar) and rose absolute are
available. Rose geranium essential oil is a cheaper alternative.*

- 50 ml/2 fl oz almond oil
- 1.5 ml/¼ tsp wheatgerm oil
- 15 drops rose essential oil
- 5 drops coriander essential oil
- 2 drops cedarwood essential oil
- glass bottle

Pour all the ingredients into a glass bottle with a stopper and gently
shake to mix. Store in a cool, dark place.

# HARMONIOUS MASSAGE OIL

*The combination of these essential oils is said to create a harmony related to the ability to love and be loved: rose is healing and sensual; sandalwood is relaxing; clary sage is euphoric and uplifting; geranium is cleansing; ginger fortifies and warms.*

- 13 drops rose essential oil
- 2 drops sandalwood essential oil
- 2 drops clary sage essential oil
- 3 drops geranium essential oil
- 3 drops ginger essential oil
- 20 ml/4 tsp jojoba oil
- 105 ml/7 tbsp unrefined sunflower oil

# AFTER-SUN SOOTHING OIL

*For anyone who has been in the sun too long without sufficient protection, this oil can moisturize and soothe tender skin, providing it is not actually burnt or broken.*

- 5 drops rose essential oil
- 5 drops chamomile essential oil
- 45 ml/3 tbsp grapeseed oil
- 45 ml/3 tbsp virgin olive oil
- 15 ml/1 tbsp wheatgerm oil

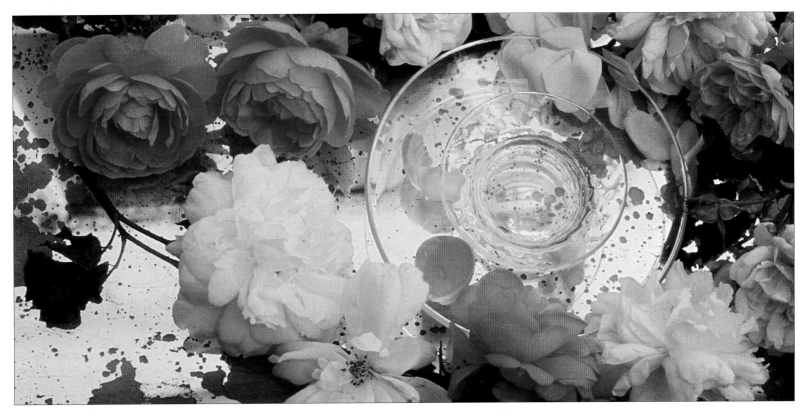

# Scented Baths and Fragrances

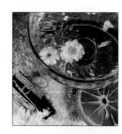

Perfumed bath oils and herbal mixtures turn bathing into something of a ceremony. Aromatic baths can have a very therapeutic effect, especially if you use essential oils to scent the water. Bath salts, milk baths and bubbles all contribute to the sense of luxury. As well as adding fragrance, these bathtime recipes include treatments to soften dry skin, soothe tired muscles, relax and

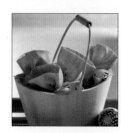

prepare you for a good night's sleep or invigorate your mind and body in preparation for the day ahead. For after the bath, try blending your own scented dusting powders and delicate colognes.

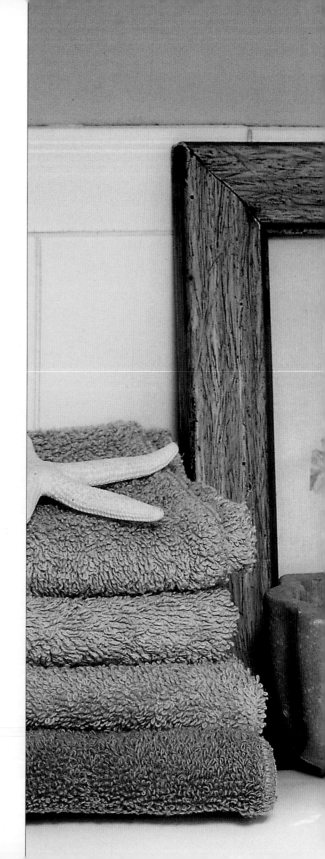

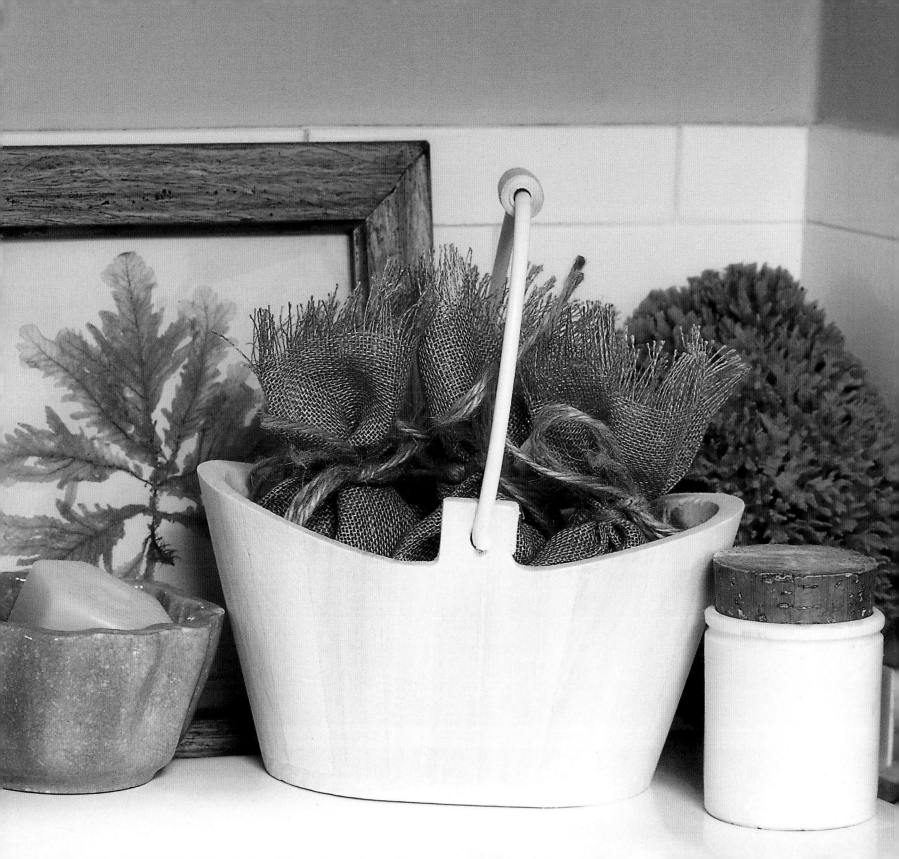

# LAVENDER AND MARJORAM BATH OIL

*A long warm bath is an excellent way of relieving the stresses and strains of a difficult day. This bath oil mixture has the added bonus of moisturizing the skin while it gently soothes away cares and troubles and relaxes your mind and body. The essential oils induce sleep. To enhance the effect, you could add a bath bag containing fresh lavender and marjoram to the water.*

- 30 ml/2 tbsp almond oil
- 7 drops lavender essential oil

- 3 drops marjoram essential oil
- small dish

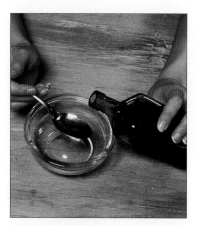

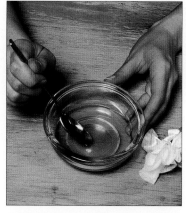

**1** Measure out all the ingredients into a small dish.

**2** Mix all the ingredients together and pour them into the bath while the water is running.

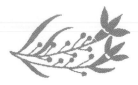

# LEMONGRASS, CORIANDER AND CLOVE BATH OIL

*As this bath will stimulate the circulation and relieve aching joints and muscles, it is ideal for anyone suffering from stiff limbs after arduous exercise. Add the oil when the bath is nearly full so that the essential oils do not evaporate before you get into the water.*

- 30 ml/2 tbsp almond oil
- small dish
- 2 drops lemon grass essential oil

- 2 drops coriander essential oil
- 2 drops clove essential oil

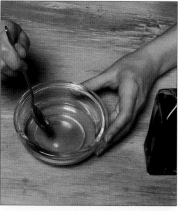

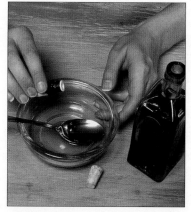

**1** Measure out the almond oil into a small dish.

**2** Slowly drop in all the essential oils. Mix all the ingredients together and pour into the bath while the water is running.

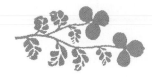

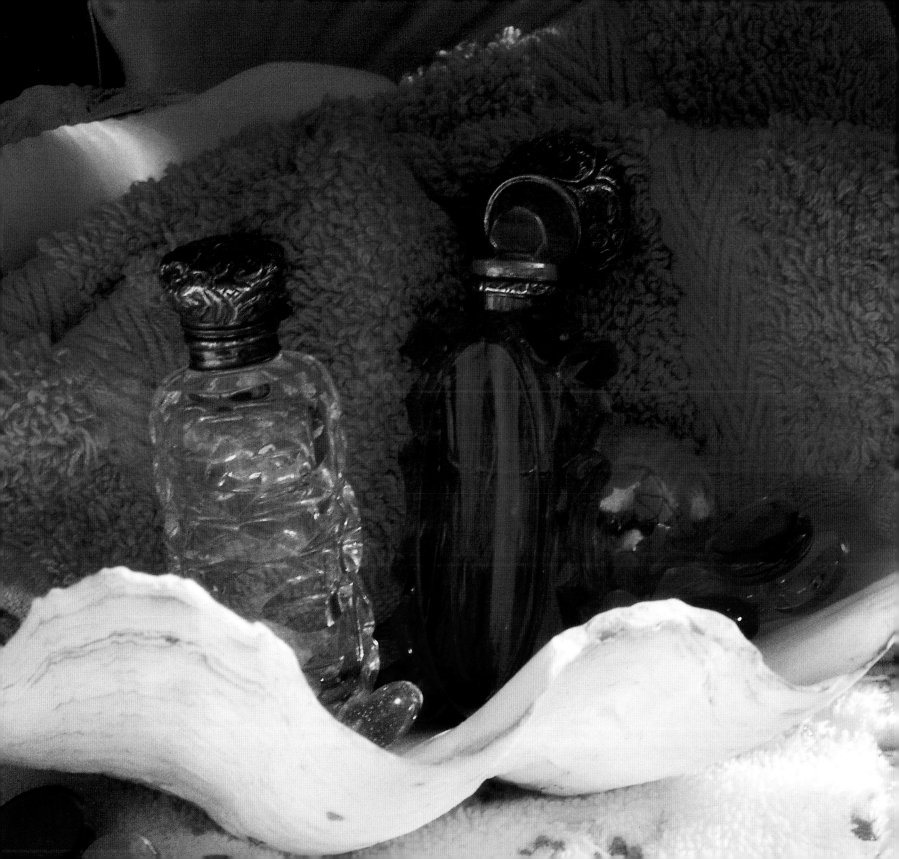

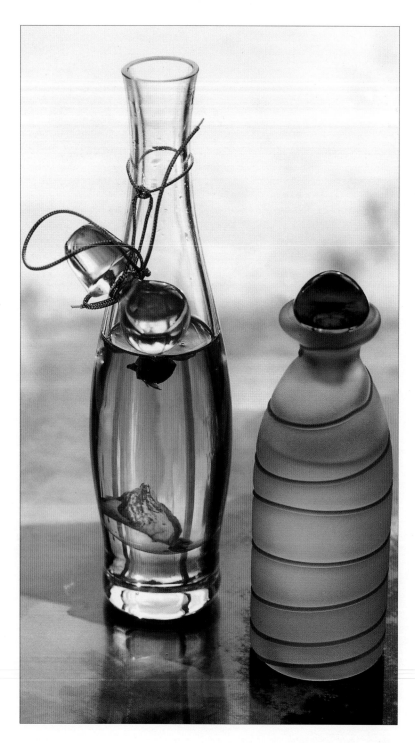

# GRAPEFRUIT AND CORIANDER BATH OIL

*Use this stimulating oil when you need reviving, especially*
*when recovering from a cold or when treating tired muscles.*
*This recipe makes enough for ten baths.*

- 100 ml/3½ fl oz/7 tbsp almond oil
- 20 ml/4 tsp wheatgerm oil

- opaque glass bottle
- 30 drops grapefruit essential oil
- 30 drops coriander essential oil

Pour the almond oil and wheatgerm oil into an opaque glass bottle, add the essential oils and gently shake to mix.

# SEDUCTIVE ROSE AND SANDALWOOD BATH OIL

*Rose essential oil may be expensive, but its scent is so powerful,*
*a little goes a long way. When combined with sandalwood oil,*
*a warm, spicy fragrance is created that lingers deliciously*
*on the skin long after the bath. Enough for ten baths.*

- 100 ml/3½ fl oz/7 tbsp almond oil
- 20 ml/4 tsp wheatgerm oil
- opaque glass bottle

- 15 drops rose essential oil
- 10 drops sandalwood essential oil

Pour the almond oil and wheatgerm oil into an opaque glass bottle. Add the essential oils and gently shake to mix.

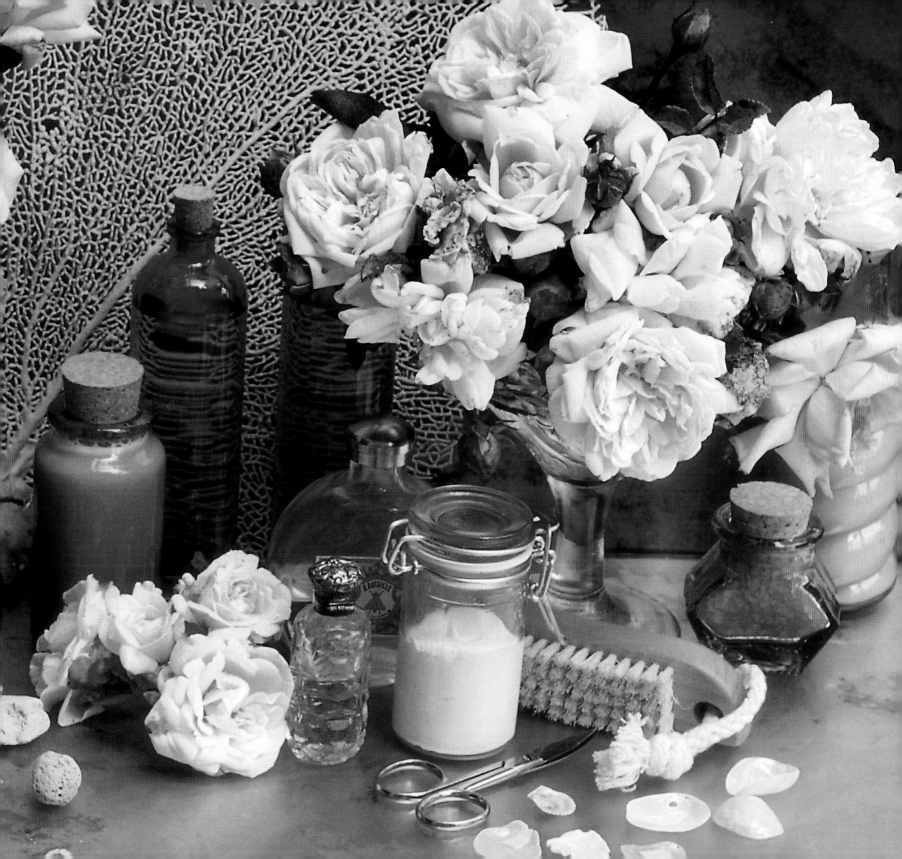

# HERBAL BATH BAGS

*Herbal bath bags can be hung over the taps so that the hot running water passes through them, releasing relaxing and comforting scents to make bathtime that much more sensual.*

- 3 x 23 cm/9 in diameter circles of muslin
- 90 ml/6 tbsp bran
- 15 ml/1 tbsp lavender flowers
- 15 ml/1 tbsp chamomile flowers
- 15 ml/1 tbsp rosemary tips
- 3 small elastic bands
- 3 m/3 yd narrow ribbon or twine

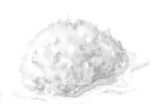

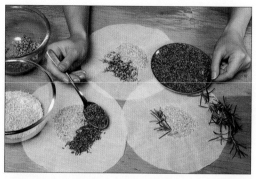

**1** Place 30 ml/2 tbsp bran in the centre of each muslin circle. Add the lavender to one bag, the chamomile to a second and the rosemary to the third.

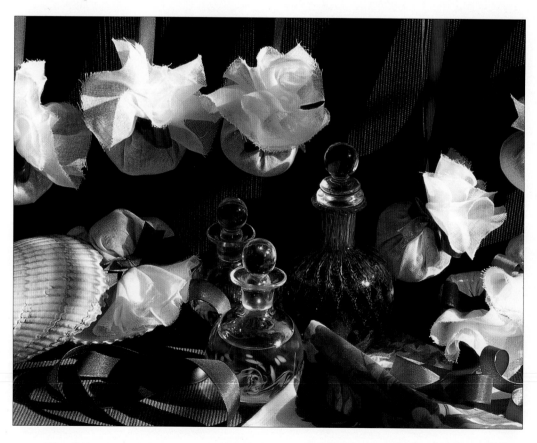

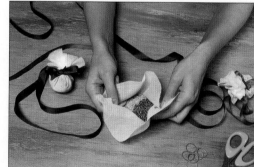

**2** Gather up each circle of material into a bundle and close it with an elastic band. Tie a length of ribbon or twine around the neck of each bag, making a loop so that the bag can be hung from the hot tap in the stream of water.

# FRAGRANT BATH BAGS

*This exotic mixture of rose petals and lavender mixed with citrus peel and bay or lemon leaves will lightly scent the bath.*
*These bags are slightly more substantial than the quickly gathered ones shown opposite, but the different fillings can be put into*
*any type of bag or pouch. Any loosely woven fabric, such as muslin or voile, will do.*

- 50 g/2 oz dried red rose petals
- 50 g/2 oz dried lavender flowers
- 25 g/1 oz dried orange and lemon peel, cut into fine ribbons
- 115 g/4 oz dried bay or lemon leaves, shredded
- 50 g/2 oz coarse oatmeal
- 8 fabric bags, 15 x 10 cm/ 6 x 4 in
- ribbon or string

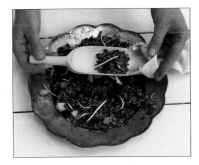

**1** Mix the filling ingredients together and fill each bag with some of the mixture.

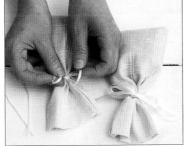

**2** Tie a large loop in the ribbon or string before securing the neck of each bag, for hanging from the tap.

## SEDUCTIVE BATH BAGS

Bath bags filled with a sleep-inducing mixture will relax you and guarantee a restful night's sleep. Make up as for Fragrant Bath Bags.

- 50 g/2 oz chamomile flowers
- 50 g/2 oz lime flowers
- 25 g/1 oz hop flowers
- 50 g/2 oz coarse oatmeal
- 8 fabric bags, 15 x 10 cm/ 6 x 4 in
- ribbon or string

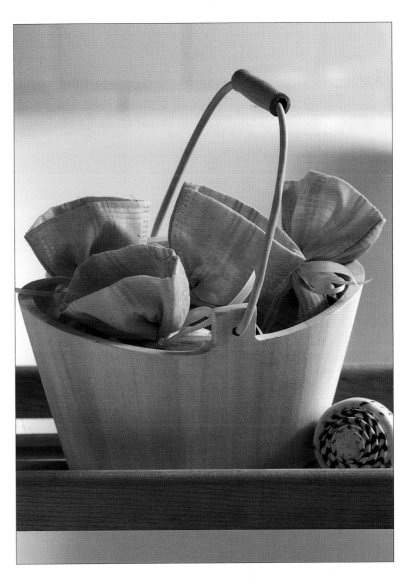

# Botanical Bath Salts

*Reviving rose bath salts are wonderfully aromatic and lift the spirits as well as scenting the skin. Calming chamomile bath salts, however, could be used before an early night. To use bath salts, just add 30 ml/2 heaped tablespoons to the running water of a moderately hot bath and immerse yourself for a maximum of 15 minutes.*

### Reviving rose bath salts

- 10 g/¼ oz dried rose petals
- pestle and mortar or electric coffee grinder
- 500 g/1¼ lb coarse sea salt
- 10 drops rose geranium essential oil
- 5 drops lavender essential oil
- 5 drops bergamot essential oil
- decorative glass jar, with close-fitting lid

### Calming chamomile bath salts

- 500 g/1¼ lb coarse sea salt
- 10 drops chamomile essential oil
- 10 drops marjoram essential oil
- 1–3 drops green food colouring
- decorative glass jar, with close-fitting lid

**1** To make the rose bath salts, grind all but a handful of the petals.

**2** Mix the ground petals into the salt, then add all the essential oils, stirring thoroughly. Fill the jar, adding a decorative layer of reserved rose petals halfway up.

**3** For the chamomile bath salts, simply mix all the ingredients together.

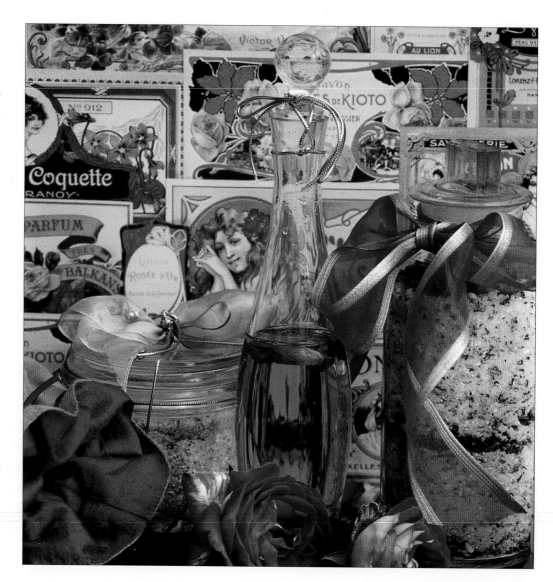

# CALMING MILK BATH

*This bath should really relax you. Chamomile and neroli are renowned for their soothing and calming properties, and are often used for treating insomnia. For a gift, present the mixture in a decorated bag accompanied by a bottle of the matching oils.*

- 120 ml/4 fl oz/ ½ cup fine sea salt
- 240 ml/8 fl oz/ 1 cup powdered milk
- 6 drops chamomile essential oil
- 12 drops neroli essential oil
- ceramic mixing bowl
- spoon
- covered container
- small calico drawstring bag
- dried chamomile or strawflower flowerheads
- dried orange slice
- fresh flowers
- grosgrain ribbon
- extra chamomile and neroli essential oils
- funnel
- empty essential oil bottle
- scrim ribbon
- matching embroidery thread

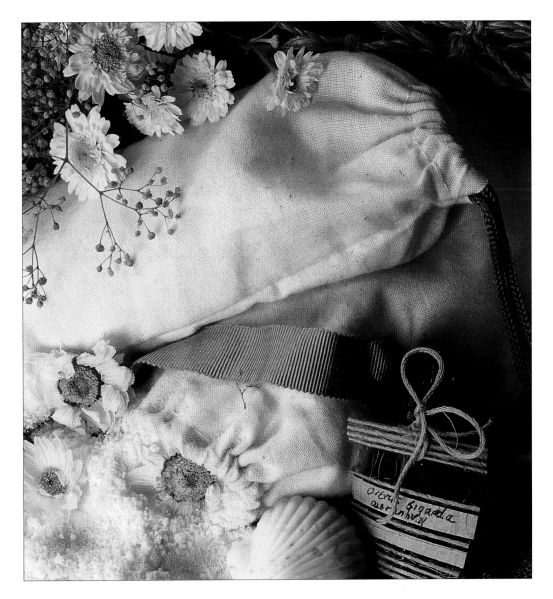

**1** Mix the sea salt, powdered milk and essential oils well. Place in a covered container and leave for 3 weeks. Decant into the calico bag, adding a few dried flowerheads. Decorate the bag with the dried orange slice, fresh flowers and grosgrain ribbon.

**2** Mix extra essential oils in the same proportions as earlier and use to fill the empty bottle. Write instructions for use on a piece of scrim ribbon and tie round the neck of the bottle, using embroidery thread.

# GRAPEFRUIT AND GINGER BUBBLES

*The stimulating combination of ginger and grapefruit makes for a refreshing bath. The inclusion of glycerine will help soften the skin and counter the effect of hard water. For a lot of bubbles, squirt an extra 15 ml/tablespoon or more into the running water.*

- 25 ml/1 fl oz/1½ tbsp glycerine, from a chemist (drugstore)
- 120 ml/4 fl oz/½ cup unscented liquid soap
- 1 drop green food colouring (optional)
- 35 drops grapefruit essential oil
- 15 drops ginger essential oil
- squeezable plastic bottle

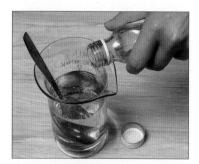

**1** Mix the glycerine into the liquid soap.

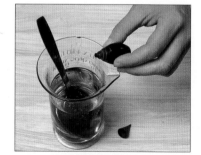

**2** Stir in the food colouring, if using.

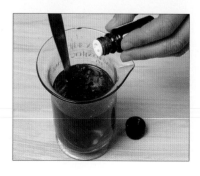

**3** Add the essential oils and stir thoroughly. Store the bubble bath in a squeezable plastic bottle.

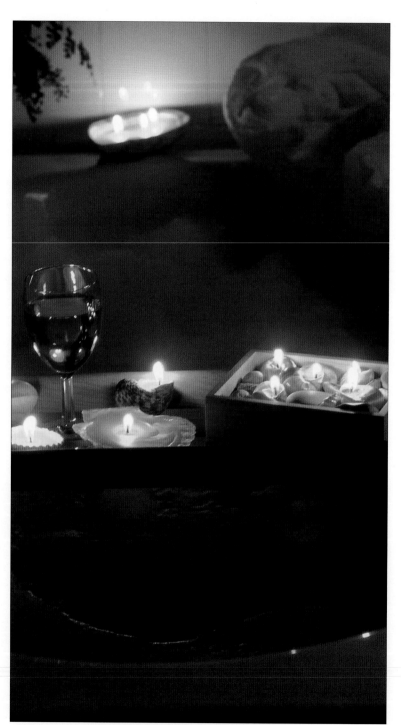

# LAVENDER BUBBLE BATH

*This delightful bubble bath is very simple to make and would be a welcome gift for friends or family.*

- 1 bunch lavender
- clean wide-necked jar, with screw top
- 1 large bottle clear organic shampoo
- 5 drops lavender essential oil
- strainer
- decorative bottle

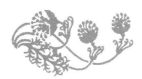

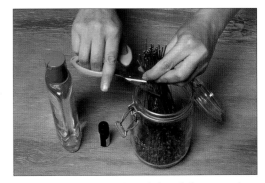

**1** Place the lavender bunch head downwards in the jar. Cut the stalks down if they are longer than the jar. Pour in the shampoo and the lavender oil.

**2** Seal the jar and place on a sunny window sill for 2–3 weeks. Shake the jar occasionally during this time.

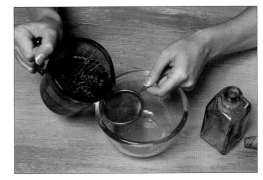

**3** Strain the liquid and pour it into a decorative bottle. Use about 15 ml/1 tbsp for each bath.

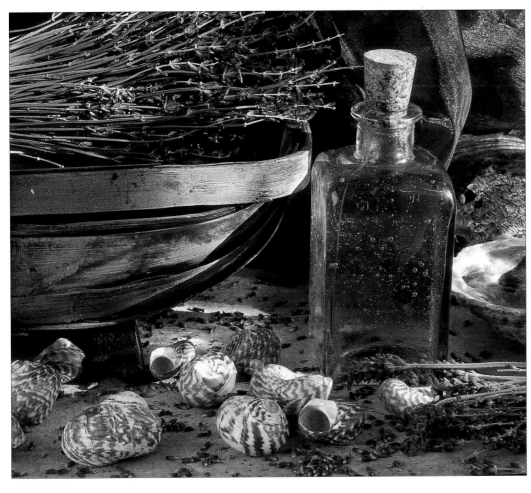

# INFUSED FLOWER BATH OIL

*The fragrance of this oil is less intense than that of a pure essential oil, but it is an excellent way of making use of an abundance of strongly scented flowers in the garden. Pick the flowers à point and dry them on kitchen paper. Repeat the infusing process with more petals until the oil is sufficiently perfumed; if you run out of petals you can add a little pure essential oil to intensify the fragrance.*

- fragrant flowers
- sterile glass jar with stopper

- cold-pressed sunflower oil
- strainer

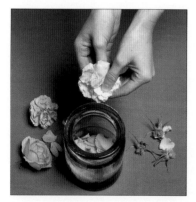

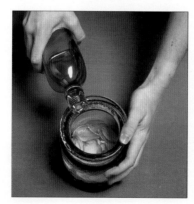

**1** Remove the petals from the flowers and pack as many as possible into the sterile glass jar.

**2** Pour over enough oil to cover the petals, then replace the stopper. Leave the jar outside in the sun for a few weeks, bringing it indoors at night. Strain and discard the flowers.

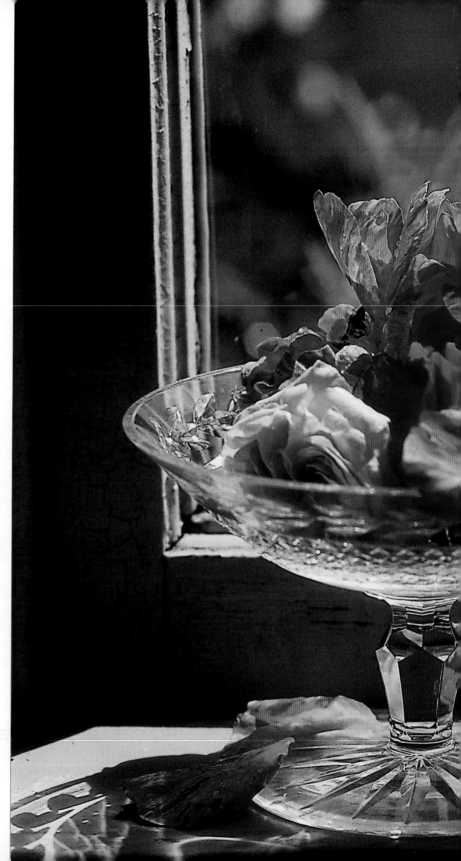

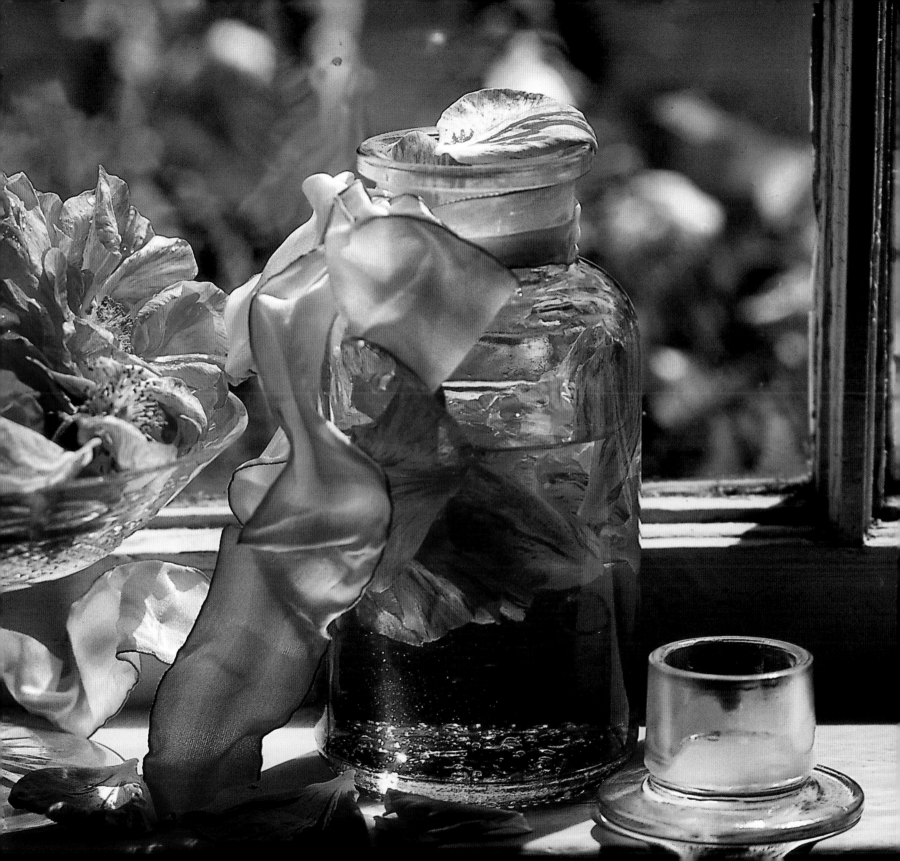

# Scented Dusting Powder

*Dusting powder can be made from scratch, using the method given below, or you can use unscented talc as a base. Single fragrance powders are the simplest to make: for every 75 ml/5 tablespoons of talc you will need 15 ml/1 tablespoon of cornflour (cornstarch), scented with 5 drops of your favourite essential oil.*
*The fragrance in the following recipe is a soft blend of lavender, coriander and geranium with a hint of fresh lemon,*

- deep mixing bowl
- 60 ml/4 tbsp white kaolin clay
- 60 ml/4 tbsp arrowroot
- 60 ml/4 tbsp cornflour (cornstarch) plus 15 ml/1 tbsp for scenting
- small bowl
- 3 drops lavender essential oil
- 3 drops coriander essential oil
- 3 drops lemon essential oil
- 3 drops geranium essential oil
- spoon
- lidded container

In a deep bowl, mix the clay and arrowroot together and add 60 ml/4 tbsp cornflour (cornstarch). Put the 15 ml/1 tbsp cornflour (cornstarch) in a separate small bowl and add the essential oils. Stir thoroughly. Add the scented flour to the larger bowl and mix. Pour the dusting powder into a decorative lidded container.

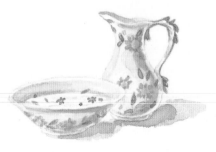

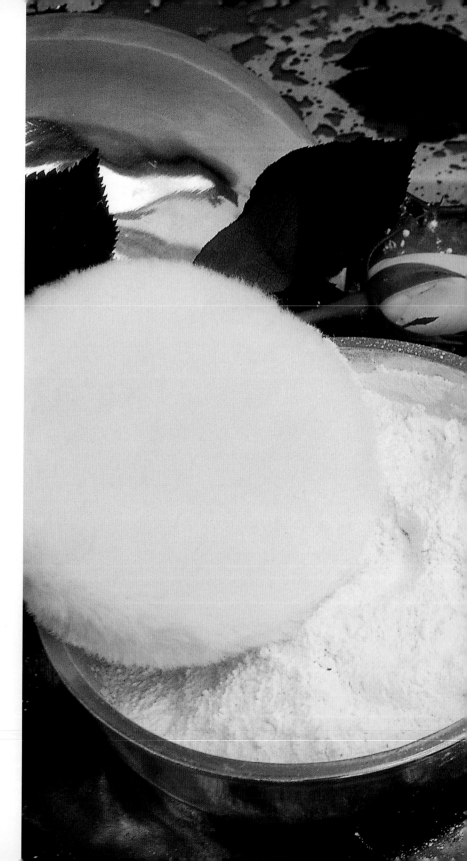

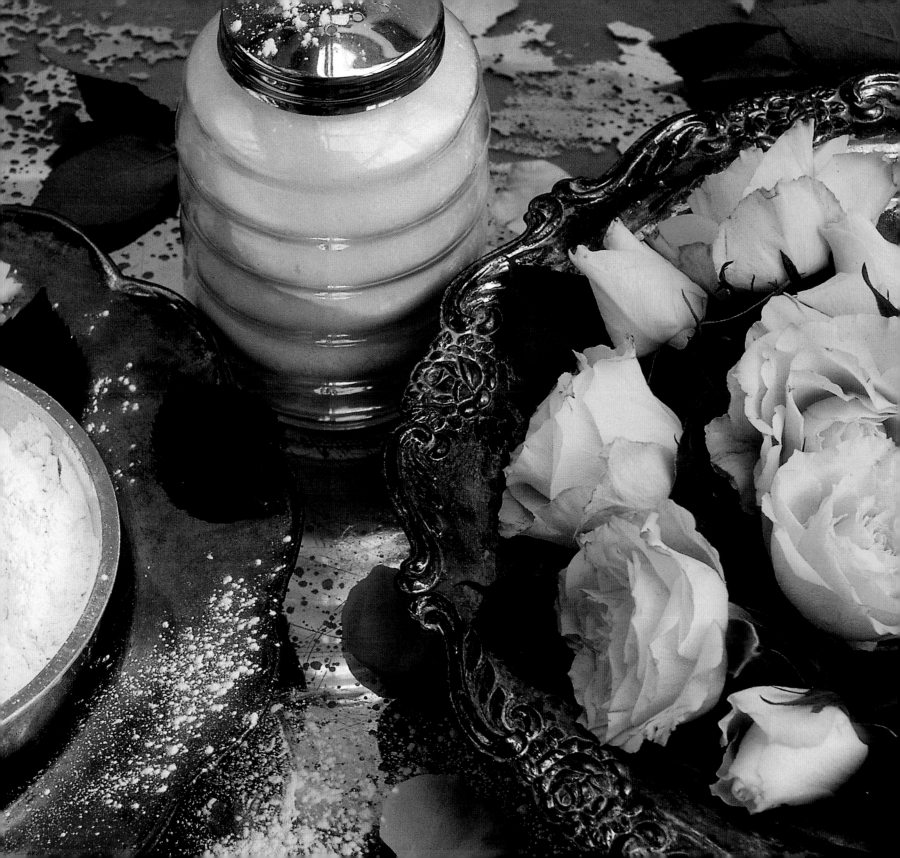

# SUMMER SCENT

*Evocative of a fragrant summer garden, this prettily scented* eau de parfum *is a delicate blend of rose, geranium and bergamot.*

- 100 ml/3½ fl oz/ 7 tbsp vodka
- glass bottle with stopper, sterilized
- 10 drops rose essential oil
- 10 drops geranium essential oil
- 50 drops bergamot essential oil
- 15 ml/1 tbsp distilled water
- 2.5 ml/½ tsp fixative tincture
- unbleached paper coffee filters
- decorative bottle or jar, with tightly fitting lid

**1** Measure the vodka into the bottle then add the essential oils. Seal, gently shake and leave to stand for 48 hours. Add the water and fixative. Replace the stopper, gently shake and leave to stand for 1 week.

**2** Shake the bottle, then strain the liquid through coffee filter papers, until the *eau de parfum* is clear and sparkling. Store in a decorative bottle or jar, ensuring that the lid is well sealed.

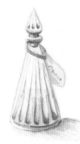

To make fixative tincture: Mix 5 ml/1 tsp powdered gum benzoin or orris root with 30 ml/2 tbsp vodka. Pour into a small screw-topped bottle and shake vigorously to mix. Leave to stand for at least 24 hours; longer is better. To use, pour off without disturbing the residue. Gum benzoin and orris root are available from companies selling pot-pourri ingredients and from herbalists.

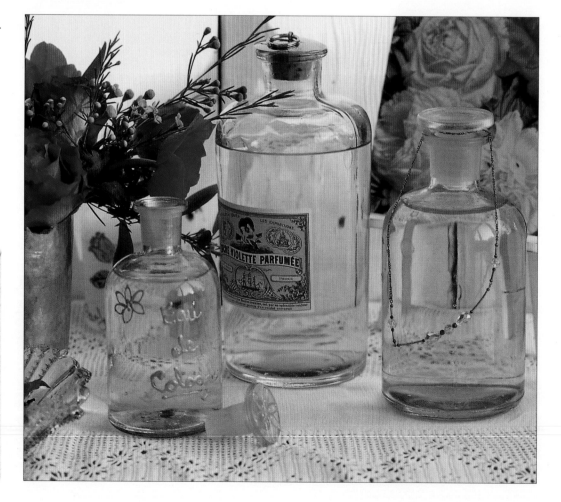

# EAU DE COLOGNE

*The fragrance of eau de Cologne is light and refreshing, perfect for an after-bath splash. Alternatively, you could keep it in an aerosol bottle in the fridge during hot weather to use as a scented cooling spray.*

- 100 ml/4 fl oz/7 tbsp vodka
- funnel, sterilized
- glass jar with stopper, sterilized
- 20 drops orange essential oil
- 10 drops bergamot essential oil
- 10 drops lavender essential oil
- 2 drops rosemary essential oil
- 50 ml/2 fl oz distilled water
- 5 ml/1 tsp fixative tincture
- unbleached paper coffee filters
- decorative bottle or jar

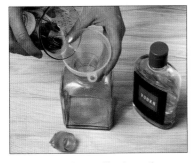

**1** Measure the vodka into the sterile jar.

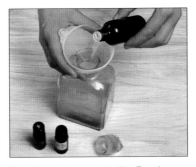

**2** Add the essential oils. Replace the stopper, gently shake to mix and leave to stand for 48 hours. Add the water and fixative tincture. Replace the stopper, shake and leave to stand for one week.

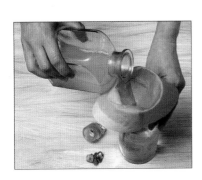

**3** Shake the bottle and then strain through a series of filter papers, until the cologne is clear and sparkling. Store in a decorative bottle or jar, ensuring that the lid seals well.

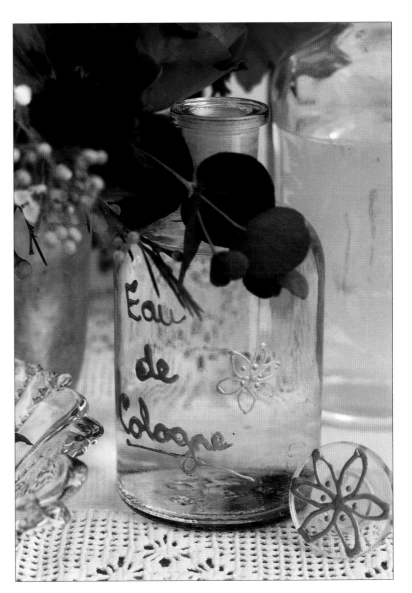

# DILL AFTERSHAVE

*Here is a fragrance recipe exclusively for men. The aftershave is best kept in the fridge so that, as well as smelling good, the cooled liquid has a bracing effect when it is applied to the skin.*

- 50 g/2 oz/¼ cup dill seed
- 15 ml/1 tbsp honey
- 600 ml/1 pint/ 2½ cups water
- saucepan
- 15 ml/1 tbsp distilled witch-hazel
- strainer
- bottle

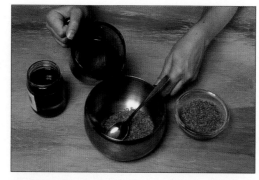

**1** Place the dill seed, honey and water in a small saucepan and bring to the boil. Simmer for about 20 minutes.

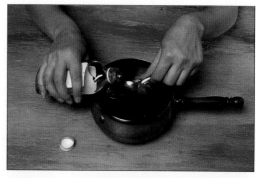

**2** Allow to cool in the pan, then add the witch-hazel. Strain the cooled mixture into a bottle.

## LAVENDER WATER

Lavender sweet water has been popular since the twelfth century. It can be splashed on as a refreshing perfume or added to a footbath at the end of a hot day to soothe tired feet.

- 350 g/12 oz/ 3 cups lavender
- saucepan
- 600 ml/1 pint/ 2½ cups water
- spoon
- strainer
- bottle
- 150 ml/¼ pint/ ⅔ cup vodka

**1** Place the lavender in a large, heavy saucepan and pour in the water and bring slowly to the boil, stirring constantly.

**2** Simmer for 10 minutes, remove from the heat and allow to cool to room temperature. Strain into a bottle and add the vodka. Shake well.

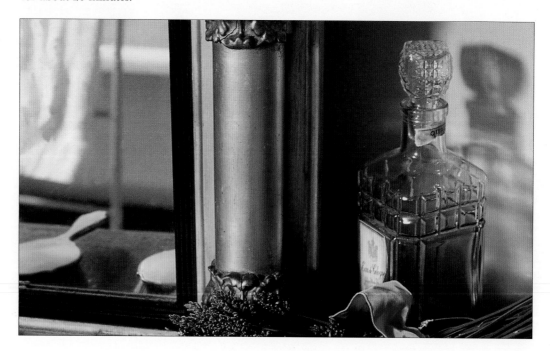

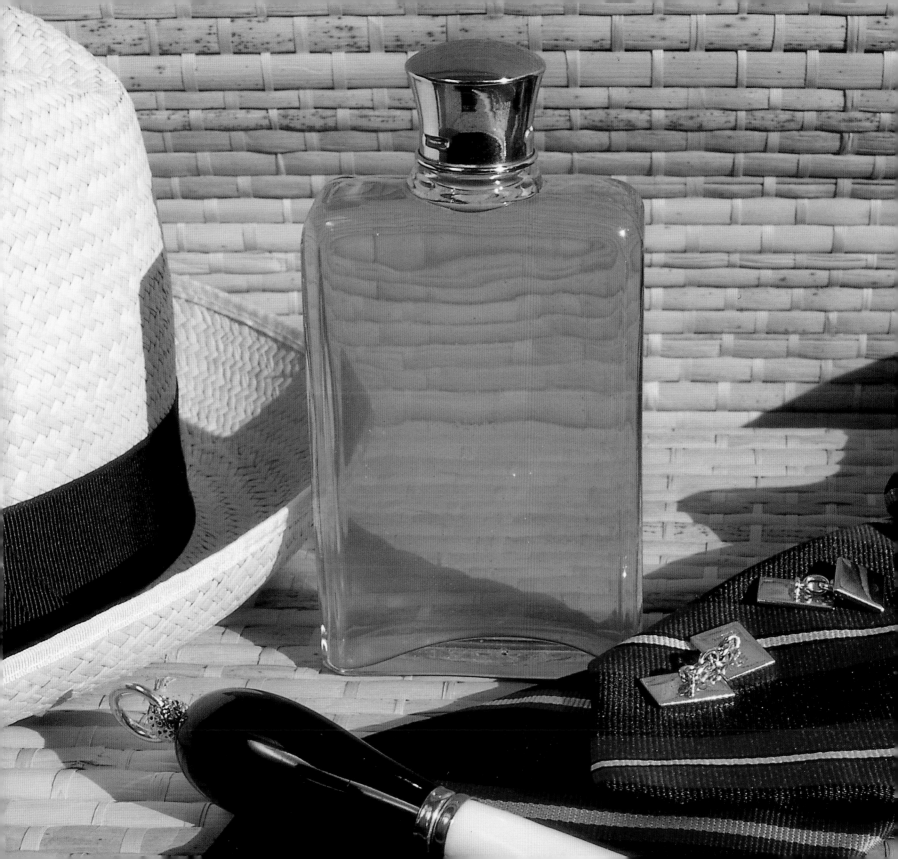

# Index

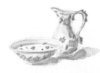
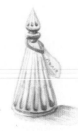